mercury

Second in the Sierra Club Battlebook Series

mercury

by Katherine and Peter Montague

Sierra Club   San Francisco • New York

Designed and produced by Charles Curtis, New York,
and printed in the United States of America by
The Guinn Company, Inc.

Contents

Foreword

Early in 1969, before assuming the editorship of *Environment* magazine, I worked on the series of articles that would appear in its May issue. This was to be a special issue devoted entirely to the problem of mercury pollution, of which we had learned from Göran Löfroth, the biochemist whose efforts to alert Sweden to the problem are described in this book. No English-language publication had yet dealt with what seemed to be a serious hazard to public health, and I was anxious to bring the contents of the forthcoming issue to the attention of the Department of Agriculture and the Food and Drug Administration.

I telephoned a number of officials in the Department of Agriculture, trying to find out to what extent mercury pollution was known and what measures were being taken to combat it. The Department of Agriculture seemed a reasonable place to begin, for I had little idea then of the extent of industrial pollution, and was most concerned about the agricultural use of mercury fungicides. Methyl mercury preparations were then—and are now—used to treat most of the wheat, corn and other grain planted in the United States to protect them from fungus attack. Research indicated very strongly that mercury compounds used this way would migrate through growing plants and would be found in the harvested crops. Swedish investigators had uncovered a disturbing pattern of concentrations of methyl mercury, the most toxic form of mercury commonly found, which could be carried from treated seed to growing plants to harvested grain. And if this grain were used to feed chickens, the chickens would excrete the mercury in their eggs, resulting in increased exposure to fanciers of the sunnyside-up.

We had quickly discovered that mercury compounds were considered so highly toxic that, despite their common use as insecticides, Department of Agriculture regulations prohibited the presence of *any* mercury residue on food crops. This is a so-called "zero tolerance," a blanket prohibition usually applied only to compounds suspected of causing cancer. Because research had shown that mercury fungicides, when applied to seeds before planting, appeared in low concentrations in the mature crop, and because mercury seed treatments of grain were almost universal, it seemed likely that essentially all of the grain being grown in the United States, and all of the animals being fed on this grain, and then used for food, were in technical violation of the USDA's regulations.

Looking back over my notes from that time, I see that I spoke to Dr. Harry Hayes, then director of the Pesticides Regulation Division of the Department of Agriculture, and a number of officials in the Food and Drug Administration's Bureau of Compliance. None of these officials expressed undue concern about mercury, none told me he believed there was a problem of food contamination aside from occasional accidental spills of mercury compounds, and none seemed to think the

Swedish problems with extensive mercury pollution were cause for alarm. The Food and Drug Administration declined to answer questions about its tests of food for mercury (the FDA is responsible for enforcing the "zero tolerance" prohibition). The Department of Agriculture was evasive, cast doubt on the results of studies which showed that mercury moved from treated seeds into grown plants, and indicated no intention of looking into the problem further.

All of these officials, and others, were sent copies of the final *Environment* articles, which pointed out some of the other sources of mercury pollution described in this book—paper, paints, and chlorine-alkali factories. Yet it was not until the poisoning of the Huckleby family in early 1970 that the tragic incidents at Minamata, Niigata, and in Sweden suddenly became relevant to the United States. As the Montagues point out, it was not surprising that the *Environment* stories provoked so little reaction—federal officials had had the same information as early as 1966. It was an old story.

Although peculiarly toxic, mercury insecticides have much in common with other agricultural chemicals. This partly explains, but does not excuse, the lack of government response to the information that most of the food in the United States was in violation of federal regulations. There is a "zero tolerance" for mercury in food—but when all food contains some mercury, this is an unenforceable regulation. There are zero tolerances for other pesticides—for instance, according to regulation, there must be no DDT at all in milk sold in interstate commerce. But all milk—and nearly everything else—contains *some* DDT. Pollution by this persistent chemical is so widespread that it has become impossible to enforce the regulations which were to have prevented the pollution in the first place.

The response to this situation on the part of federal agencies has been, unhappily, predictable. It has been to ignore the regulations which were being violated. In the case of DDT, which is now ubiquitous in the environment, the responsible agencies accepted what seemed to be an irreducible level of pollution as "background," and only took action when DDT levels, in milk for instance, were severely higher than the average. This approach has required the Food and Drug Administration to establish a series of informal "action levels," concentrations of pesticides above the "normal" background level which would stimulate it to action. In a series of interagency agreements, this approach became formalized, and the "zero tolerance" regulations were all but abandoned.

In the case of mercury, the situation was complicated by the presence of some mercury of genuinely natural origin in all foodstuffs. The problem of identifying added mercury from human activities was a serious one, although there is little evidence it was dealt with seriously. Until the sensational revelations of high mercury levels in fish were made by Canadian biologists, the FDA did not even have an action level for mercury —and still has none for foods other than fish.

In the 1950s, radioactive fallout from nuclear weapons tests became the first pollution problem to command national attention. Here was the classic pattern of small doses of toxic material being administered to millions of people—in fact, to the whole population of the world. Large doses of radiation were known to be harmful, but the amount of radiation exposure received by any one person was small. There was difficulty in defining the risk this sort of broad, low-level exposure represented. And then, too, there was "natural background" radiation, the steady universal exposure we all receive from cosmic rays and radioactive chemicals found naturally in the environment. Man-made fallout, except in areas of great concentration, was generally small compared to natural radiation exposure.

As fallout levels rose (and public consternation with them) the standards for safe exposure were approached. The Federal Radiation Council, the agency established to set federal policy in radiation matters, responded by raising the allowable limits to make room for the actual exposures. Years later, the Food and Drug Administration would take the same approach to pesticides in food.

The unfortunate fact about radiation, however, is that there can be no truly "safe" exposures—any amount of radiation is damaging to some extent, if administered to a large enough number of people. This is presumably true of natural radiation, also, which is probably the cause of at least some naturally occurring cancers and birth defects. Permissible levels of exposure have always been acknowledged *not* to be safety standards, but rather judgments of how much damage from radiation is acceptable in exchange for the benefits to be derived from a particular source of radiation.

Methyl mercury has much in common with radiation. There is growing evidence that even very small exposures, far less than those permitted by existing standards, can do damage to the brain and perhaps to the reproductive cells. There is a certain background level of natural mercury, which is converted to the methyl mercury form by bacteria, and it is possible that this natural material contributes to the burden of illness that each generation carries. "Permissible levels" of mercury in food are therefore not guarantees of safety, they are limitations on damage already being done. The degree of damage we will permit is a matter of how valuable we feel the activities which produce mercury contamination are, and how costly it would be to clean them up.

In Sweden, the banning of methyl mercury compounds in agriculture probably resulted in lower costs for the farmer. Although some other mercury compounds judged to be less harmful to the environment are still in use, they are applied much more sparingly than previously. Crop yields have not declined as a result. It seems, in fact, that methyl mercury seed dressings for grain were used far in excess of what would have had real value in agriculture, and that the resulting pollution problem was simply unnecessary.

In 1969, even though the Swedish ban had already been in effect for some time, the U.S. Department of Agriculture informed me that there was no substitute for methyl mercury compounds. I was told that the banning of methyl mercury compounds was impossible. More recently the department has, after all, moved to ban methyl mercury compounds, and despite legal delays, will probably succeed in doing so. To my knowledge, there has been no sudden discovery of a substitute unknown in 1969.

More mercury is discharged to the air in the United States than is received by its waters or farmlands. As the Montagues point out, coal contains some mercury, and when it is burned in power plants, the mercury is released to the air. Mercury entering the air from power plants and municipal incinerators probably far overshadows other sources of industrial mercury pollution. The high levels of mercury found in bird feathers from as early as 1900 probably originated in the process of burning coal.

Controlling mercury contamination should not be difficult. For these problems to persist means only that we are balancing the profit of some individuals and businesses against the public good, and finding the private profits more important. Mercury-based chlorine-alkali plants, for example, are no longer being built in Sweden, and that country has not visibly suffered as a consequence. But a ban on such plants in this country seems not to have occurred to federal officials, even though perfectly satisfactory means for making chlorine and caustic soda without mercury are available.

How many other environmental problems stem from trivial or unnecessary industrial habits? The bulk of our DDT has always been used on southern cotton—to combat the boll weevil—yet it is not effective for this purpose and probably never was. Now excessive pesticide use is beginning to result in damage to cotton and other crops, particularly in the southwest and west, and yet every move to restrict pesticide use is opposed by their manufacturers. After years of attack by citizens' groups, the manufacturers of nuclear power plants have finally begun to add devices that restrict emissions of radiation to levels far below those permitted by federal regulations, and still greater improvements could be made, at trivial cost (so-called zero release systems add less than one percent to the cost of a nuclear power plant).

When are we going to insist that Detroit spend our money on nonpolluting automobiles instead of on yearly style changes? That the packaging industry turn its attention from manipulating the consumer to protecting his health from food-borne disease, now reaching epidemic proportions? That federal subsidies be given toward the recycling of materials instead of toward more mining and lumbering? That agriculture be turned away from the wasteful use of fertilizers on crops stimulated to greater growth on smaller acreages to take advantage of federal payments? That railroads be improved and supersonic aircraft be forgotten? That the endless proliferation of highways, which produce their own congestion, be halted?

None of this means any retreat from an industrialized society, or a decline in our standard of living. On the contrary, all of these measures to preserve our health and the environment are also measures which would mean more useful economic activity, more goods that are desired, and a better way of life even in terms of our consumer culture.

The mercury problem, as described in this excellent book by the Montagues, stands for the environmental crisis as a whole. There is no need to continue licensing our industries to poison our water and food, to blight the land and cloud the air, out of a long-held but mistaken idea that this damage is somehow inevitable. Only ignorance and special interest can defend such a view any longer. To clean up the environment means only to insist that industry serve our purposes as well as its own. The result should, in the long run, mean a better life for everyone.

Sheldon Novick

Under the shed at the Golden West Seed Company in Texico, New Mexico, the rats that night gnawed through the sacks of sweepings. And the grain and seeds sifted down from the sacks and powdered the earth. Some of the seeds were brown as the earth, but others were unnaturally pink. So the rats suppered, never suspecting it would be one of their last, even as the hogs in the Huckleby pen in faraway Alamogordo would never suspect that the feed trucked to them from under the same shed had been pinked by a panogen mercury fungicide dressing.

And least suspicious of all were the Hucklebys themselves, who enjoyed fried pork.

1. Quicksilver:

Anatomy of a poison

The ancients called it quicksilver, after its bright color
and fast, elusive ways. Mercury was a plaything, then.
No more. Now men mine mercury to purify other
metals, to kill germs, to prevent mildew, to protect
seeds, to complement dental fillings, to measure the temperature of the human body. And all of these seem
good. Yet through such uses, directly or indirectly, men
have released into the environment new compounds of
mercury that could ultimately—if they have not done so
already—visit long-lasting harm on humanity itself.

Of the harmful effects of mercury too little is known.
But *great* potential harm is suspected. Still, the uses of
mercury increase while the warnings grow more omi-
nous and urgent.

A century ago, when fur hats were in fashion, mercury was used to improve fur's felting qualities. Workers who became afflicted with persistent tremors in-

spired no great public concern. They simply inspired the phrase "mad as a hatter." But today the phrase-makers are silent, for the presence of mercury in the human diet—on the dinner plate, if you will—is no joking matter. Poisonous mercury, it appears, is turning up everywhere, especially in food fish. Though the various government agencies responsible for monitoring mercury levels apparently cannot agree on how much of the poison man may safely ingest—or, indeed, on whether he should ingest any at all—the fact remains that mercury, the pollutant, is too much with us in the 1970s. Its presence, as Senator Philip Hart (D-Michigan) pointed out after listening to two days' testimony by specialists, may well constitute "the greatest environmental crisis in our history."

"A national disaster," said Ralph Nader.

Many scientists agree that mercury does indeed present a considerable hazard. *Science* magazine, for example, the official publication of the American Association for the Advancement of Science, has branded mercury pollution a "substantial hazard" and "long-enduring problem." In one editorial, *Science* editor Philip Abelson warned:

> Of particular significance is methyl mercury, a highly toxic substance that causes neurological damage, produces chromosomal aberrations, and has teratogenic effects. It is mainly in this form that mercury is found in food fishes.

Science's crisp terminology cloaks a catalogue of physiological horrors: *Neurological damage*—meaning destruction of brain cells, a burning out of the body's delicate control links. *Chromosomal aberrations*—genetic damage which may not surface for three, four,

five generations, unpredictable structural damage to
any of the body's parts or systems, cancer. *Teratogenic
effects*—literally, "monster-creating effects," birth defects, damage to the growing fetus while it's still inside
the mother's womb, inexplicable seizures, severe mental
retardation.

In its natural metal form, mercury is not highly toxic. In fact, in an attempted suicide a person once actually injected two grams of metallic mercury directly into
his veins without ill effect. The mercury merely formed
a puddle in the right side of his heart. So it is not pure
quicksilver that poses a hazard, but rather the inorganic and organic compounds derived from the basic metal.

Inorganic mercury is generally divided into three
main subgroups. First, elemental mercury vapor. In
this form mercury is quite dangerous, especially because it can be ingested so readily through the lungs.
The second group of inorganic compounds includes
mercurous and mercuric salts, which find wide industrial and medical use. They are not as toxic as the
organic mercury compounds; still, before barbiturates,
drinking a gram of mercuric chloride was the most
common way for Americans to commit suicide. A third
kind of inorganic mercury is found chemically bound to
proteins.

Organic mercury compounds are highly toxic and are
used in slimicides and fungicides, mildew-killers,
germ-proofing sprays, crab-grass eradicators, among
other products. There are three major classes of organic compounds: phenyl mercury, methoxyethyl mercury
and alkyl mercury. Of them all, the most deadly are the
alkyl compounds, ethyl and methyl mercury. The latter

has been recognized as a special hazard to people since at least 1880. A very small amount of methyl mercury can cause severe disintegration in the human nervous system.

Metallic mercury is an element, No. 80 on the periodic table, one of the basic, irreducible building blocks of planet earth. Thus, though the forms and chemical combinations of mercury may change, and though mercury may shift location about the planet, still the total amount of mercury in the earth must always remain constant.

Several natural systems—the wind, the rain, volcanic disturbances—continually distribute mercury throughout the environment. In addition to being the only metal that remains liquid at normal earth-surface temperatures, mercury also evaporates, just as water does, changing into a gaseous vapor. In its vaporous state mercury travels wherever the winds blow. But wherever conditions of temperature and barometric pressure coincide appropriately with mercury's own vapor pressure, the vapor abruptly changes back into the silver liquid metal and returns to earth (or the sea) as "dry fallout," as it is known to geochemists.

In addition, rain continually washes mercury vapor out of the atmosphere. Some of the mercury in rain water remains waterborne, ending up in the sea (which now contains an estimated 50 million metric tons of elemental mercury). The remainder of it enters the upper two inches of the earth's crust, where it very soon binds itself chemically to plant fibers, soil constituents and microorganisms. Wherever mercury enters water or soil, some of it inevitably ends up in food chains.

Thus, the crust of planet earth is alive with quicksilver as the substance drifts from place to place, concentrating now in this particular pocket, later in another.

Throughout the earth's crust the concentration of mercury seems to average about 60 parts per billion (ppb). This means you would have to dig up and refine a billion pounds of earth materials to get 60 pounds of virgin mercury. Of course mercury is not distributed evenly over the earth's crust and there are some spots, almost always near volcanic activity, where mercury appears in high concentrations. One ore in particular, red cinnabar, contains 13.8 percent sulphur by weight and 86.2 percent pure virgin mercury. (See Appendix, Table of Weights and Measures.)

Pure metallic mercury is obtained by mining and refining cinnabar, which usually appears not in pure form but in combination with other minerals and rocks. Mercury mined in the United States in 1969, for example, averaged a return of five pounds of mercury for each ton of earth materials. The refining process is relatively simple. Ore is heated inside a closed container. The resulting mercury vapors are drawn off, cooled down in a condenser, collected and put into flasks holding 76 pounds of metal, ready for sale. On the New York wholesale market a flask will bring an average of $508, or $6.68 per pound.

Approximately 110 mines produce mercury in the United States, but 11 mines account for upward of 77 percent of all U.S. mercury production. The important mercury-mine states are: California ($9.3 million, value of 1969 production), Nevada ($4.1 million), Idaho ($511,000). Oregon, Alaska, Arizona and Texas also produce substantial quantities. The total dollar value of the 2,231,360 pounds of virgin mercury mined in the United States in 1969 was $14,828,000.

U.S. mercury *consumption* that year far outstripped U.S. *production.* In addition to consuming virgin U.S. mercury, industry also dipped into three other sources.

First, the United States in 1969 imported 1,155,732 pounds of mercury from Bolivia, Canada, Ghana, Italy, Mexico, Spain, England and Yugoslavia. Second, some 18 percent of all mercury consumed in 1969 came from recycling—redistillation of mercury captured from defunct mercury vapor (steam) boilers, for example. Third, in recent years the Atomic Energy Commission has been selling thousands of flasks of mercury (supplying up to 23 percent of total U.S. consumption needs per year). The AEC since World War II has held an unspecified, large stockpile of mercury for unspecified, large purposes. Policy shifts a few years ago resulted in much of the AEC's mercury flowing back onto the U.S. market.

About 80 companies, most of them located in the eastern United States, accounted for 96 percent of the nation's mercury consumption in 1969 (a quantity representing 27 percent of total world production). These industries are involved in the production of chlorine and caustic soda, electrical fixtures, paints, catalysts, pesticides and pharmaceuticals, among other products. All together, there are an estimated 3,000 industrial uses of mercury; and while some uses have declined in recent years, others have multiplied rapidly. The utilization of mercury as a cathode in the electrolytic preparation of chlorine and caustic soda, for example, has more than tripled since 1959 and now requires more than 1.5 million pounds of the metal each year. (See Appendix, The Industrial Uses of Mercury.)

The U.S. Geological Survey often speaks of mercury "leaking" from American factories, and industrialists invariably speak of mercury "escaping" from the sewage systems that their own company engineers designed. The truth is, American industry has dumped at least 40 million pounds of mercury into the nation's waterways since 1930, passing on to the consumer both the cost of the wasted resource as well as the pollution. Indeed, the 40-million-pound figure may be a conservative estimate. Since 1900, industry has "consumed" at least 165 million pounds of mercury. This is according to the Bureau of Mines' "consumption" figures.

There are other important sources of mercury pollution. Combustion of fossil fuels, for example, releases huge quantities of mercury into the environment annually. Somewhere between 275 and 1,800 tons of mercury pour from the 550 million tons of coal burned each year in the United States. Other pollution sources are tin, zinc, copper and gold smelters, which release large quantities of mercury into the air. Diaper services, commercial laundries and the manufacturers of a thousand pastes, glues, adhesives and sizing compounds use mercury, and sometimes dump it. The manufacture of explosives—one of the fastest-growing industries in the United States—employs undisclosed amounts of mercury annually.

No one apparently has a very clear idea of where all this mercury is going. Only one thing seems certain: It doesn't "go away." It's still around in the biosphere somewhere. In aquatic environments, mercury compounds remain active for 10 to 100 years.

To begin to measure industrial pollution, one must first ascertain the natural amounts of mercury present in unpolluted environments. The Geological Survey and the Oak Ridge Laboratory have compiled such data.

• Soil seems to average concentrations of about 100 ppb mercury, but soils in the western United States seem to average about 500 ppb.

• Rocks contain mercury in concentrations ranging from about 5 ppb to about 10,000 ppb—and in some cases even higher.

• Unpolluted air contains between 3 and 9 nanograms of mercury per cubic meter of air. One nanogram is one billionth (1/1,000,000,000) of a gram, or 0.035/1,000,000,000 of an ounce. One cubic meter equals about 1-1/3 cubic yards. Nanograms per cubic meter is a measure of the amount of elemental mercury vapor present in a volume of air, and it is expressed ng/m³—nanograms per meter cubed, or per cubic meter.

• The air over the ocean seems to contain less mercury than the air over land. Twenty miles out at sea the background level is 0.6 to 0.7 ng/m³.

• Rain water averages 0.01 ppb as a background level. Rain water that has fallen through polluted urban air may contain up to 0.48 ppb, a significant increase.

• Sea water seems to contain mercury at a background concentration ranging from 0.03 ppb to 2.0 ppb. The background level in fresh water is 0.1 ppb.

• In fresh-water fish the background level is higher,

being measured in parts per million (ppm), not parts per billion. The background level in fresh-water fish living in unpolluted waters is 0.2 ppm or less.

These, then, are the figures against which mercury pollution must be measured. As we shall soon see, what has been measured already in some locations is alarming.

"It looks all right to me," said one of Ernest Huckleby's two friends. "And we ain't going to eat it ourselves anyway."

The man from Golden West Seed Company shook his head. "I don't know," he said. "If it were me, I wouldn't feed it to no hog."

Still, though some of the sweepings were pink, they were also free. And Ernest Huckleby and his friends, who had borrowed a flatbed truck and driven the 200 miles from Alamogordo when they heard some feed was being given away, weren't about to turn around and go back empty. "We'll take it," said one of Huckleby's friends.

They took five and a half tons. Back in Alamogordo, they mixed the seeds and the grain with regular slops and fed it to their hogs. "I don't see that it can hurt," said one of the men. "Do you?"

Ernest Huckleby didn't answer. He was watching the big fat boar, figuring the time left till butchering.

2. Minamata:

A case of the kibyo

Minamata is a quiet town on the southwest coast of Kyushu, the most southerly of the main Japanese islands. Its two principal industries—at least in the early 1950s—were fishing and the manufacture of chemicals. Fishing predominated. One could surmise as much by observing the fishermen's nets hung to dry in the afternoon sun, or by considering the large number of cats in town, fat and content from the offal of the fishermen's daily catch, and the crows, which also shared in the feast. As for the chemical factory, there was nothing of importance to note, except, perhaps, for the channel that carried its effluents directly into Minamata Bay.

In April 1953, Minamata was visited by a series of strange occurrences. It began with a cat—a wild, leaping, screeching cat that dashed suddenly past a group of playing children. Pursuing the animal, the children ran down to the beach and stood in open-mouthed wonder as it plunged headlong into the sea. The cat struggled briefly in the waves, went under, surfaced, then sank, drowning, dead.

"*Kibyo*," said one of the watchers from the shore. *Strange illness.*

Yes, said another. The cat surely was a victim of a *kibyo*.

Then the crows went crazy. As the Tanaka family children gathered to greet their father returning from his work at sea, they saw crows falling from the sky. A bird would plummet straight down, catch itself short of impact with the ground, fly falteringly upward, only to fall once more. Very strange, everyone who saw the falling crows agreed. *Kibyo.*

The following day the youngest member of the Tanaka family complained of soreness in several places and of a curious constriction of vision that made the world look as if it existed at the end of a tunnel. Next, the father began to complain of dizziness and numbness in his fingers and his lips. He fell down when he tried to walk. Progressively, he and his six-year-old son lost the ability to control their bodies at all. They both soon lost use of their minds as well and entered a hospital where they had to be restrained in their mad ravings. Within two months, both died.

For a distance of nearly four kilometers down the coast from the town, family after family reported severe, irreversible illness in one or more members. And during the next nine years, of some 110 individuals who developed symptoms, 36 died. The afflicted survivors of the *kibyo* suffered debilitating damage to their nervous systems, including blindness and deafness.

Japanese health authorities were baffled, but since

cats had died of the disease, and almost all of the afflicted humans were from families of fishermen, they immediately looked to fish for the cause.

Forty families suffered from Minamata disease between 1953 and 1956. Of these, 25 families ate fish or shellfish from Minamata Bay every day. The other 15 families ate fish or shellfish from the bay at least two or three times a week. An analysis of silt from the bay bottom revealed that the area was polluted by a large factory, by the very same chemical factory that dumped its wastes into Minamata Bay.

Doctors and public health authorities began to suspect metals poisoning when autopsies on four of the dead revealed intestinal necrosis. In addition, a particular brain lesion in one victim led researchers to believe the metal manganese might be involved. Other evidence led them to suspect the rarer elements selenium or thallium.

In 1957, researchers produced Minamata disease experimentally in cats by feeding them fish from Minamata Bay. This merely confirmed what public health authorities had already suspected. In fact, authorities had closed Minamata Bay to commercial fishing as of December 1956, after 42 cases of the disease were reported earlier that year.

In 1958, while on a visit to Japan's Kumamoto University, Dr. Douglas McAlpine, a physician from Glasgow, Scotland, suggested that methyl mercury compounds could cause some of the symptoms of Minamata disease. Subsequently, two Kumamoto investigators in 1961 experimentally produced Minamata disease in cats by orally administering methyl mercury compounds. Then they went to the big chemical factory, the only one in the little town, and inquired about the use of mercury in its industrial processes. The Glasgow physician, Dr. Douglas McAlpine, and a colleague from Kumamoto University, Dr. Shukuro Araki, had investigated the Minamata factory three years earlier, in 1958. They were told at the time that the factory manufactured fertilizer and that its principal effluents were ammonium sulfate, ammonium and calcium phosphate, sulphuric acid, carbide and nylon, an odd list at best. But now a closer investigation showed that the factory had also been producing the very popular plastic polyvinyl chloride (PVC), using mercury as a catalyst. And in the factory's effluents, the investigators found strong traces of mercuric chloride—one of the inorganic salts.

How did the factory's less harmful inorganic mercuric salts change into the highly poisonous methyl mercury associated with Minamata disease? The Kumamoto investigators later theorized, after analysis of the plant's effluent, that biological organisms—bacteria, or tiny animals—methylated the mercuric chloride in their bodies and then excreted the deadly poison. From the organisms, the poison then spread throughout Minamata Bay.

The investigation now turned to determining how much fish containing how much methyl mercury had caused the disease. This was a complicated problem. By the time testing got underway in earnest in 1961, conditions in Minamata Bay had changed radically. For one thing, the amount of mercury in the factory's effluent had increased steadily between 1949, when its PVC production was 60 tons, and 1959, when its PVC production was up to 18,000 tons. In addition, the factory in 1958 had rechanneled its effluent away from the bay and into the Minamata River near the point where it

enters the open sea. Thus, when investigators checked
mercury levels in the sediment and sea water of the
bay, they could not be sure what their measurements
meant. They were measuring residues at least three
years old.

In any event, mercury concentrations in silt near the
plant reached 2,010,000 ppb (parts per billion). In the
water of Minamata Bay itself, investigators reported
finding mercury concentrations ranging between 1.6
and 3.6 ppb. As we have noted, the normal range for
sea water is 0.03 ppb to 2.0 ppb, so Minamata Bay even
in 1961 was significantly polluted.

The more important question regarding contamination levels in fish wasn't resolved until a second outbreak of poisonings occurred at Niigata, Japan, in
1965. All together, 120 persons at Niigata reported
having one of the symptoms of Minamata disease:
numbness in the fingers or toes, numbness around the
mouth, or constriction of the visual field. Twenty-six
persons complained of all three symptoms, so Japanese
health records show only 26 official cases of Minamata
disease at Niigata in 1965. Of these, five died.

The Niigata poisonings provided important experimental data. These data showed that full-fledged Minamata disease resulted from eating fish 0.5 to 3.0 times
per day. The average serving of fish at a meal was generally estimated at either 150 or 200 grams. And the
type of fish eaten was found to be contaminated at levels between 5,000 ppb and 20,000 ppb, wet weight.

"The Niigata poisonings . . . clearly demonstrated
that the consumption of fish containing 5 to 6 ppm
[5,000 to 6,000 ppb] daily would probably be lethal,"
writes Dr. J. M. Wood of the University of Illinois.

Most important of all, the Niigata poisonings confirmed what the Minamata outbreak had only suggested: that methyl mercury is teratogenic, that it can cause birth defects if eaten by pregnant women. For at Minamata and Niigata together, a total of 22 children were born defective. In most cases, they were born to women who had eaten mercury-contaminated fish during pregnancy but who had not developed symptoms of Minamata disease themselves. This, of course, indicated that the fetus is more susceptible to damage by methyl mercury than is the adult human.

Autopsies on children afflicted by fetal Minamata disease showed the characteristic damage to brain cells. Methyl mercury seems to dissolve brain cells, leaving in their place empty cavities filled with inert fluid. In addition, methyl mercury burns out the farthest links of the nervous system, in the fingers and toes, causing the characteristic numbness that victims usually experience.

Worst of all, the Niigata poisonings seemed to confirm yet another possibility: that methyl mercury in fish can cause genetic damage in humans, destroy chromosomes, or even cause production of an abnormal number of chromosomes in human sex cells.

Inside the pen, the hog lay on the hot ground, pawing the air.

"Huckleby's hog got the blind staggers," said one of the men.

"Sure got something. And two others dead already."

"Lucky they not all sick though," said the first man.

"Not yet, anyway."

The prostrate hog shuddered then. A fly landed on its open eye.

"Huckleby's lucky," said the first man. "He butchered that other big one yesterday. Bet his family going to enjoy that meat."

3. Fungicide:

The seeds of death

When German chemical entrepreneurs discovered in 1914 that organic mercury compounds could be marketed as fungicides, few dreamed that agricultural mercurials would soon support a booming industry. By 1968 world consumption had reached 4,724,977 pounds. Farmers are easily persuaded by chemical industry salesmen that organomercurials increase crop yields.

Applied to seeds before planting, or to the young plants themselves, the organomercurials are said to protect against such diverse enemies as bunt, root rot, covered smut, net blotch, dry rot and blast.

Thus, since 1940, mercury compounds have come into worldwide use on wheat, barley, oats, rye, maize (corn), rice, sorghum, linseed, millet, cotton, flax, apples, pears, apricots, cherries, peaches, almonds, walnuts, strawberries, cucumbers, watermelons, pumpkins, squash and potatoes. But when the United States finally enacted its first pesticide regulations in 1947, mercury compounds were placed in the "zero tolerance" category. This meant that, by law, no mercury residues could be found on food shipped interstate—*no* mercury residues, none. Yet organomercurials are still used by some U.S. farmers.

Sweden was also sluggish in recognizing the inherent hazards of mercury on the farm. There in the early 1950s conservationists noted decreasing populations of seed-eating birds—pheasant, partridge, pigeon, finch. Simultaneously, they encountered increasing numbers of bird carcasses around the Swedish countryside. But bird watchers in those days weren't taken seriously—and Swedish health authorities easily brushed off reports of ecologic damage from agricultural mercurials. The evidence, they said, was insufficient.

Consequently two young radiobiologists, Dr. Gören Löfroth and Dr. Carl Rosén, decided they would systematically survey the Swedish environment for signs of the damage officials refused to recognize. Teams of radiologists, biologists and chemists—led by Westermark, Sjöstrand, Christell and others—developed and refined an analytic technique called neutron activation analysis for measuring extremely small amounts of mercury—down to .01 ppb—in biological samples. Löfroth and Rosén and their colleagues collected data on birds and mercury for several years. They repeatedly documented high levels—up to 200,000 ppb—of mercury in the livers of birds.

By 1960 predatory birds, which feed upon the seed-eaters, came to the attention of the mercury investigators. Buzzards, goshawks, sparrow hawks, owls and eagles were showing up with elevated levels of mercury. In

1962 the Swedish Central Seed Testing Institute recommended that "lowered doses" of methyl mercury be used.

Soon other specialists joined the investigation. In 1963 Dr. Gunnel Westöö revealed preliminary findings in her broad sample of Swedish hens' eggs: mercury, she found, averaged 29 ppb. (By way of contrast, the background level for uncontaminated hens' eggs in the United States then was about 3 ppb.)

A Swedish sample of 200 wild birds in 1964 revealed mercury concentrations exceeding 2,000 ppb in 51 percent of all birds. That same year, the Swedish Plant Protection Institute (Växskyddsanstalten) recommended cutting mercury concentrations in seed dressing by 50 percent. It was no great victory for the conservationists, but it was a beginning.

In early 1965 Dr. Torbjörn Westermark and Dr. Alf Johnels authoritatively reported elevated mercury concentrations in the edible portions of fish taken from several Swedish lakes. Here was startling news. And later that year Dr. Westöö reported finding that the mercury compound in eggs, meat *and* fish was methyl mercury, the most toxic mercury compound known. The Japanese had, of course, been right.

By the fall of 1965 Swedish health authorities decided that perhaps they had been wrong all along, that mercury *was* a problem. A national information conference convened rapidly in Stockholm that September. With much attendant publicity, specialists sketched in monograph after monograph a convincing and worrisome picture of environmental pollution by mercury.

Convinced by the conference that methyl mercury was polluting the environment from *at least* agricultural sources, Swedish authorities acted swiftly. Under Royal Ordinance the Swedish Plant Protection Institute severely restricted the use of methyl mercury in agriculture, effective November 1, 1965. As of February 1, 1966, the Swedish Poison and Pesticides Board refused continued registration of any alkylmercury compounds for agricultural uses. On the same date, the board denied phenylmercury acetate continued registration for use in the Swedish paper industry, effective October 1, 1967.

So great was Swedish concern at the extent of environmental pollution by mercury that an international symposium was convened just four months later—in January, 1966—to spread information throughout the world scientific community. Curiously, the Japanese were not invited.

U.S. authorities attended the 1966 conference. Inexplicably, they failed to hear the alarm.

On December 4, 1969, Ernestine Huckleby, 8, fell from the monkey bar at school and was sent home. She complained vaguely of pains. That night, as she undressed for bed, her mother, Lois, noticed that she was having particular difficulty with buttons. The little girl's fingers were fumbling.

The next morning Ernestine stumbled and fell as she came to the breakfast table. She tried to get up. And fell again.

At the Tularosa Clinic, Dr. E. J. Klump ordered Ernestine Huckleby into an El Paso, Texas, hospital immediately. A pediatrician there said at first that it looked to him like spinal meningitis.

4. Warnings:

Through rosy glasses

The international conference in Stockholm revealed significant mercury pollution throughout most of Sweden. Not surprisingly, the evidence suggested that quicksilver pollution was a recent and growing phenomenon, the byproduct of industrialization. Using birds from museums, Swedish analysts demonstrated that mercury levels in bird feathers, 1960 to 1965, exceeded mercury levels, 1860 to 1865, by a factor of 10. Around the turn of the century, it was reported, levels in Swedish wildlife began rising, with the biggest increases occurring after 1940. But bird kills weren't the only dangers from methyl mercury discussed at the 1966 conference. Several researchers described studies of Swedish fresh-water fish that showed high levels of mercury—levels as high as those found at the scene of the two Japanese disasters. The edible portions of pike *(Esox lucius)* showed mercury levels as high as 20,000 ppb and the mercury was reported to be almost 100 percent methyl mercury, the deadliest kind.

Various U.S. executive departments and the President's Office of Science and Technology sent five representatives to Stockholm to monitor proceedings of the meeting. The Office of Science and Technology is intimately associated with the Federal Council on Science and Technology, the agency charged with bringing important scientific questions to all departments simultaneously for action. Representing the United States were: Dr. R. W. Weiger of the U.S. Public Health Service (under the Department of Health, Education and Welfare) ; Dr. F. N. Ward of the U.S. Geological Survey (Interior Department) ; Dr. E. H. Dustman, director of Patuxent (Maryland) Wildlife Research Center (Interior Department) ; Dr. Kenneth C. Walker (Agriculture Department) ; and Dr. John L. Buckley for the President's Office of Science and Technology.

According to Drs. Dustman, Buckley and Walker, the Swedish picture in 1966 gave no indication that environmental pollution by mercury might be a problem in the United States. Dr. Buckley recalls that mercury failed to alarm American participants in the symposium because Sweden's problem stemmed from only two apparent sources: methyl mercury seed dressings used in agriculture, and methyl mercury slimicides used in the paper industry.

The American paper industry had been forced by an FDA ruling in 1964 to cut its use of mercury slimicide. The FDA ruled that no mercury residues whatever could appear in paper food packages. Since paper manufacturers couldn't tell which batches of pulp would make up which final products, the FDA ruling eliminated mercury compounds completely from many American mills. Mercury used by the pulp and paper industry dropped from 215,156 pounds in 1963 to just 47,044 pounds in 1965. Thus, explains Dr. Buckley, only Sweden's *agricultural* problem with mercury seemed likely to become a U.S. problem.

A communication circulated to symposium participants before opening day—"Background information: a survey of the situation in Sweden," by the distinguished ecologist, Dr. Bengt Lundholm—did, however, describe other industrial sources of mercury. In fact, Dr. Lundholm said the chlorine-caustic soda industry (also called the chlor-alkali industry), not the paper industry, is Sweden's biggest industrial user of mercury. Anyone looking at the U.S. chlorine-caustic soda industry in 1966 would have found a revealing parallel: our biggest single user of mercury in America in 1966 was the chlor-alkali industry.

In his summary of the Swedish situation, Dr. Lundholm described total Swedish mercury usage in industry and agriculture. He then predicted that some 20 metric tons of mercury (44,092 pounds) would pollute Swedish air and water during 1966.

During 1965, according to the U.S. Bureau of Mines, U.S. industry and agriculture consumed 5,590,560 pounds of mercury. According to U.S. Geological Survey estimates, probably 25 percent of this leaked to the American environment. If U.S. mercury pollution in 1966 remained at 1965 levels, then 1,397,640 pounds (634 metric tons) of mercury would have reached the American environment that year as man-made pollution.

As U.S. officials returned home, certain that America had no mercury problem, the pollution here actually was exceeding that in Sweden by a factor of 32. Somehow, American officials had missed the message.

The Swedish information conference spurred research in other countries, but not in the United States. According to Dr. Dustman, director of the Interior Department's Patuxent Wildlife Research Center, the Bureau of Sport Fisheries and Wildlife sampled a few pheasant and a few fish along the Atlantic seaboard in late 1966. Negative results discouraged further efforts. It apparently did not occur to anyone that U.S. techniques for "looking" weren't very sophisticated.

In Canada, a different story was developing. A University of Toronto chemist, Dr. Robert Jervis, had visited both Sweden and Japan in 1965 when so much disturbing new information surfaced. Jervis had worked with the highly sensitive analytic technique called neutron activation analysis and was well prepared to begin searching the environment for mercury at trace levels. By October, 1966, Jervis had written the Canadian Department of National Health and Welfare, Ottawa, warning of possible environmental pollution by mercury and requesting a study grant. When the grant was approved he began work. Throughout 1967 and 1968 Canadian health and game officials watched Swedish research closely. The Fisheries Research Board of Canada and the Food and Drug Directorate of the Canadian Department of Health and Welfare both began translating and publishing short articles on mercury pollution, written by Swedish specialists. These translations became available at irregular intervals throughout 1967 and 1968.

A key question left unanswered by the 1966 confer-

ence was, where was the methyl mercury coming from?
Methyl mercury seed dressings contaminated birds,
but what was the source of mercury contamination in
fish? There were sources of mercury pollution in Swedish waters—paper mills and chlor-alkali plants—but
they discharged inorganic mercury, the relatively non-
toxic kind. Fish taken from polluted waters contained
the deadly methyl mercury. Here was the same puzzle
Minamata investigators had first faced.

In 1966, without proof but acting on strong suspicion, Westermark, Johnels and Olsson published their
opinion that methyl mercury could be created by bacterial action within anaerobic (oxygen-free) ecosystems—such as in mud on lake bottoms. This theory of
biological methylation had been put into print as early
as 1964 by the Japanese investigator, T. Kondo, in the
publication of the Pharmaceutical Society of Japan, but
Swedish investigators seem not to have known it. It
was a provocative thesis. If it proved correct, every industrial user of mercury dumping his wastes into a
stream or lake might be providing raw material for
creation of large amounts of one of nature's deadliest
poisons. Then, in 1967, Dr. Arne Jernelöv and Dr.
Sören Jensen reported results (published in 1968)
showing that anaerobes in mud at lake bottoms, for example, can methylate inorganic mercury. How it happened they could not yet explain. But an explanation
wasn't long in coming.

In 1967 Dr. Carl Rosén, radiobiologist from Stockholm University, spent the year teaching at the University of Illinois. There he met the vitamin B researcher, Dr. J. M. Wood. Urged by Rosén, Wood
applied for a $30,000 grant from the National Science

Foundation to experiment with methylation of inorganic mercury in anaerobic ecosystems. NSF awarded the grant and in short order Wood, Rosén and their co-worker Kennedy, illuminated the findings of Jensen and Jernelöv. The puzzle was finally solved. Now it was confirmed that microorganisms in mud metabolise metallic and inorganic mercury, excreting them as the highly poisonous methyl mercury. No matter what form mercury takes when it is dumped into storm sewer, stream or lake, biological systems can slowly convert some unknown portion of it into the deadly poison, methyl mercury. Then, by a long-understood process called organic complexing, the soluble methyl mercury spreads systematically throughout the aquatic environment into which it has been introduced, collecting and concentrating in various biological pockets. It appears not only throughout the water itself and in the microorganisms that take it up first but eventually in other plants, then in fish, finally in birds and people.

This information from Wood, Rosén and Kennedy should have alerted the American public health and scientific establishments. However, when the three researchers submitted their findings to *Science,* publication of the American Association for the Advancement of Science, the manuscript was rejected. At least one outside reader reportedly told the editors of *Science* that the manuscript wasn't worth printing.

In May, 1967, the World Health Organization, the Food and Agriculture Organization and the International Atomic Energy Agency (IAEA) jointly sponsored a discussion in Amsterdam on the subject, "Mercury Contamination in Man and his Environment." The participants issued a report of their findings in which

they urged *all industrialized nations* to monitor their
environments for mercury pollution. Reversing a previous WHO recommendation of 1963 (that the maximum permissible level of contamination in food for humans be set at 50 ppb) the World Health Organization
in 1967 reported that:

Modern studies of the distribution of mercury in
human foods and beverages and in human tissues
in different environments and at different ages are
urgently required. Until the results of such studies are available it is not possible to set meaningful
maximum permissible limits to dietary intakes of
this element. Every effort should therefore be
made to control and reduce this form of contamination of the environment and consequently of
food.

In July, 1967, the Battelle Memorial Institute, a
2,500-man privately endowed think-tank with headquarters in Columbus, Ohio, completed a two-year contract study for the U.S. Public Health Service
(USPHS) to design an overview system for evaluat-
ing the public health hazards of chemicals in the environment. The institute's two-volume report contained a
38-page appendix on mercury. After describing industrial uses of mercury, the Battelle study devoted one
page to "environmental hazards." The institute reported:

Mercury may naturally accumulate in some part of
our food chain. Minamata Bay in Japan appeared
to be an example in which industrial wastes containing mercury had been discharged into a bay
and mercury had accumulated in fish eaten by people. More recently, a Japanese report indicates

that a bacterial species can concentrate environmental mercury in its protoplasm 100,000,000 times. [The institute's report at this point cites a source which doesn't pertain.] . . . In Sweden mercury has been found in birds, fish and other footstuffs. . . .

[T]he increase of mercury in foods due to the use of pesticides has been of concern, especially in Sweden. There are numerous reports of mercury accumulation in plants treated with mercurial pesticides.

The report's gross understatement that the Minamata incident *appeared* to be a case of industrial poisoning through human food-chain contamination probably fostered the official lethargy with which the report was greeted.

The Battelle paper wasn't the first worrisome report on mercury that the U.S. Public Health Service appeared to ignore. In 1960, while visiting Japan, Dr. Leonard T. Kurland of the National Institute of Neurological Diseases and Blindness, Public Health Service, Bethesda, Maryland, examined patients suffering from Minamata disease. Upon returning to the United States, Dr. Kurland investigated shellfish from Galveston Bay, Texas, and Chesapeake Bay, Maryland. In 1960 he reported finding mercury in oysters in Chesapeake Bay at levels as high as 1,000 ppb and mercury in mussels as high as 2,000 ppb.

The mercury pollution story first broke in the American press March 11, 1968, when McGraw-Hill's *Air and Water News* described the Swedish problem briefly:

Mercury pollution. . .has been one of the most worrisome pollution problems in Sweden. Though the use of mercury compounds has now been completely stopped [This was an erroneous statement in 1968 and still isn't true today—mercury is still in use in Swedish industry and its control remains voluntary, not statutory.—K&PM], the mercury remains in the water and is deemed dangerous to humans because it is absorbed by the fish. The mercury content of some Swedish water bodies is so high that commercial fishing in them has been forbidden.

Two months later, Food and Drug Administration (FDA) officials in the Department of Health, Education and Welfare (HEW) learned about mercury at a Netherlands conference of the Codex Alimentarius Commission, a U.N.-affiliated food standards group. According to Richard Ronk, mercury project officer in FDA's office of compliance, Swedish scientists at the conference discussed mercury pollution with FDA officials. And at that time, FDA considered monitoring the environment for mercury, especially in fish. But scarcity of funds and low per-capita consumption of fish in America led FDA officials to postpone their program. In addition, says Ronk, the National Shellfish Sanitation Program, which tests shellfish from the nation's estuaries for contamination, wasn't yet revealing any danger from mercury.

Now that high mercury levels have been found in many fresh-water streams, FDA officials realize shellfish are not a good indication of ambient mercury levels. But in 1968, when the decision had to be made whether to test the nation's water for mercury, shellfish were thought to reflect pollution conditions accurately for all serious contaminants, including the heavy metals.

In the fall of 1968, Wood, Rosén and Kennedy published their important findings in the British journal *Nature,* with the following recommendations:

Methyl mercury could be formed by both enzymatic and non-enzymatic reactions, thus making this cumulative poison available for incorporation into various organisms in the aquatic environment, and secondarily into terrestrial predators. The cumulative nature of mercury poisoning can be titrated [analyzed] in fish. The extensive survey performed in Sweden has prompted legislation on the use of organomercurials in agriculture in addition to close control of mercury pollution [from industry]. Similarly in Japan legislation was brought into effect after the Minamata disaster. We feel that the example set by these two countries should be followed elsewhere before concentrations of mercury reach a point where methyl mercury is being titrated in humans as well as fish.

A few weeks later, writing in the British *New Scientist* under the title, "The Menace of Mercury," Dr. Arne Jernelöv reiterated his finding that the major source of Swedish methyl mercury was industrial, not agricultural. Jernelöv then asked—and answered—the question, "Are Sweden and Japan the only countries with high amounts of mercury in fish? It seems likely that the situation will be more or less similar in most other industrialized countries . . ."

In the world's most highly industrialized country, the public health establishment meanwhile kept its head firmly in the sand.

Now it was Amos Huckleby, 14, who complained of pains in his neck. Overnight, the boy's vision deteriorated. He could see only pinpoints of light in the very center of everything, as if he were peering down a long tunnel. His jaw went slack.

The day after Christmas, Dorothy Jean Huckleby, 20, likewise developed ataxia. And on December 27, Ernestine, who had been discharged from the hospital undiagnosed, returned to El Paso. Now she was blind. In the afternoon she lapsed into a comatose state. She would remain in that condition for eight months.

5. Thresholds:

Brain damage

Nowhere in the United States was the mercury alarm sounded as loud and clear as in the May 1969 issue of *Environment* magazine, which was devoted entirely to the subject of environmental contamination by quicksilver. In three articles, the magazine described the Japanese disasters, catalogued the Swedish experience, and openly speculated that mercury would be discovered throughout the American environment by anyone who took the trouble to look for it. Apparently, no one did.

The pathology of mercury was, by this time, quite well understood in terms of both the individual and the environment. Wildlife poisonings by mercury seed-dressings, for example, were considered much more serious than mere body-counts of birds might indicate. Dr. Hans-Jörgen Hansen of the Swedish National Veterinary Institute has compared bird counts to "an iceberg, hiding most of its mass—the subclinical test cases—below the surface." Hansen lists other hidden environmental effects of mercury—"decreased productive ability among birds, lowered resistance to other poisons (such as aldrin, a pesticide) but also to infections and parasites. Mercurials also doubtless mean lowered resistance to stress of any kind and finally a decreased ability to avoid enemies. Wildlife deaths of these sorts won't be counted as mercury poisonings, but mercury will be partly responsible for them." As has been pointed out, Swedish mercury investigators discovered many difficulties distinguishing effects of mercury pollution from those of pollution by organochlorine pesticides (the so-called hard or persistent pesticides—DDT, aldrin, endrin and a half dozen others). Since organochlorine pollution is now widespread in the world, it becomes increasingly difficult to determine precisely which environmental damage to ascribe to which chemical pollutant.

In some cases, however, the specific environmental effects of mercury are known. For example, there is the effect of mercury compounds on plant growth, especially in aquatic environments. Phytoplankton are microscopic plants that drift loose in the water. As they manufacture chlorophyll through their photosynthetic mechanisms, phytoplankton produce most of the earth's organic material and most of the oxygen for the earth's atmosphere. Obviously, any interference with the chemistry of phytoplankton can have extremely serious consequences throughout the biosphere. If phytoplankton were discouraged from doing their daily duty, life on earth would cease.

Organic mercury—including the kind that is manufactured by bacteria when there is a little inorganic

mercury in mud and no oxygen present—has been pin-
pointed in laboratory experiments as a strong inhibitor
of phytoplankton activity. In November, 1970, writing
in *Science,* three University of Florida researchers reported laboratory experiments with three different organic compounds. of mercury added in measured
amounts to water containing phytoplankton. Here is
Science's own abstract of the Florida research: "Concentrations of organomercurial fungicides as low as 0.1
part per billion in water reduced photosynthesis and
growth in laboratory cultures of one species of marine
diatom and several natural phytoplankton communities
from Florida lakes." Photosynthetic activity reduced at
concentrations as low as one-tenth of one part per billion is extremely somber information. It takes very little
industrial pollution to bring background levels up to
more than 0.1 ppb in large bodies of water and begin a
decrease in phytoplankton activity.

The threat to phytoplankton received specific recogni-
tion in the widely circulated Mrak Report *(Report of
the* [HEW] *Secretary's Commission on Pesticides and
Their Relationship to Environmental Health).* Named
after the commission's chairman, Dr. Emil M. Mrak,
chancellor emeritus, University of California at Davis,
the Mrak Report in December, 1969, brought together
the findings of 143 experts from government, industry
and universities, plus a staff of 100 specialists, assessing
the environmental effects of pesticides. The Mrak Report remains the most authoritative single work available on pesticide pollution, and of phytoplankton it observed:

Drifting plant cells in natural waters carry on a
large portion of the photosynthesis on the earth's

surface. They synthesize most of the earth's organic material, producing most of the oxygen of the atmosphere, and participate in other essential ways in the chemical cycles of the biosphere. *Evidence that pesticides may significantly reduce such processes is unusually important.* (Emphasis added.)

In addition to producing the earth's oxygen, phytoplankton stand at the bottom of the earth's food chains. It is through phytoplankton that mercury begins moving outward through the food chain of an aquatic environment:

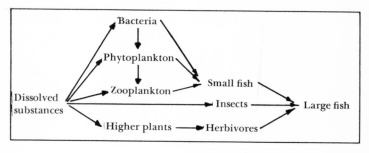

Courtesy of U.S. Geological Survey.

Mercury dumped into water may form a variety of compounds with other chemicals that happen to be found in the same locale. If sulphur is present in the environment, for example, mercury may form a sulfide compound, which is slightly soluble. Then the sulfide would dissolve slowly and move about with the currents. Methyl mercury, the extreme poison which is created by bacteria in the absence of oxygen, is both soluble and volatile, so it spreads quite readily through the water and also escapes into the air. Phytoplankton take mercury into their own bodies directly from the surrounding water and pass the mercury on to the zooplankton (mi-

croscopic animals) which eat them. Small fish eat the
zooplankton, large fish eat the small fish, and other predators eat the large fish. From water to fish flesh the
mercury increasingly concentrates itself. A pike concentrates mercury in its body in the ratio of approximately
3,000 to one, comparing flesh concentrations to ambient
water concentrations.

Mercury can concentrate in fish because fish excrete
mercury slowly. And mercury has a "half-life" of 200
days in fresh-water fish. If a fish takes in a certain
amount of mercury today, half of that mercury will remain in its body at the end of 200 days; and half of the
remaining mercury will stay in the fish for another 200
days. Any new mercury added to the fish during the 200
days simply increases its total body burden. Thus, mercury is called a "cumulative" poison—one that circulates
unchanged for a long time in the blood.

Methyl mercury is noted primarily for its ability to
dissolve brain cells and attack other parts of the central
nervous system. The question is, how much mercury
does it take to harm the brain? This raises another question: Is there a threshold level for mercury, a level
below which there is no observable damage? Dr. Alan
Hinman at the federal Center for Disease Control at
Atlanta believes there is no threshold. "Only one brain
cell at a time may be killed," he says, "but eventually they
add up." Dr. Göran Löfroth, completing a report in
March, 1969, entitled "Methyl Mercury: A Review of
Health Hazards and Side Effects Associated with the
Emission of Mercury Compounds into Natural Systems,"
also discussed the question of a threshold level. Can a
person eat a certain amount of methyl mercury in fish

and have absolutely no damage show up in clinical investigation? Dr. Löfroth answered:

As to the *gross* clinical symptoms one can state that
a threshold mechanism is operating. This threshold
mechanism is, however, not due to a methylmercury
threshold but to a threshold in the number of damaged brain cells. After damage of one or a few cells,
other cells may take over—the net result showing
up as *no* effect in the clinical investigation.

On this same subject, a professor of medicine at Washington University (St. Louis) Medical School, Dr. Neville Grant, wrote in the May 1969 *Environment:*

From the nature of the injury in the nerve tissue
caused by mercury poisoning, it is clear that the absence of symptoms does not mean the absence of
damage. The damage may go on out of sight for
some years and may be of great significance as the
poisoned person ages. The malfunction of the nerve
cells damaged by mercury may at first be compen-
sated for by viable neighbors, but as these normal
neighbor cells are removed by the aging process,
neurological abnormalities could become markedly
enhanced.

Methyl mercury is excreted slowly from the human
body. The so-called half-life of mercury in humans is 70
days. When a person eats a quantity of mercury, his
body retains half of that mercury for 70 days, and so on
(as in the case of a fish). There is plenty of time for the
poison to circulate throughout the body in the blood-
stream, doing its work, concentrating in particular
spots: the cortex of the brain, for example. Laboratory
experiments on humans have shown that 15 to 20 per-

cent of the body's entire methyl mercury content will lodge in the brain.

In pregnant women, methyl mercury passes readily through the placental barrier, entering the fetus. The Swedish physician and industrial hygienist, Dr. Stig Tejning, who has studied the toxicology of mercury compounds for 15 years, reports that the bloodstreams of newborn infants contain mercury concentrations averaging 28 percent higher than concentrations in the bloodstreams of the mothers. In addition to collecting excessive mercury, the fetus also concentrates the mercury in its brain, especially in its cortex. Even when a pregnant woman eats fish contaminated at levels insufficient to damage much of her own brain, she may be damaging the brain of her unborn child. The effects, as demonstrated by the Minamata poisonings, leave no doubt about the potency of mercury as a poison, especially to unborn infants.

Between 1955 and 1960, 17 children born near Minamata, Japan, were reported suffering from infantile cerebral palsy. They had all been born to mothers who ate some fish but who did not develop the disease (though some of the women did report numbness in the fingers or around the lips). Examinations of two of these children revealed clinical evidence of fetal Minamata disease. At the age of 16 months the first case, a female, "had spastic paralysis of all extremities with exaggerated tendon reflexes. She was unable to perform any useful movements, such as turning over in her sleep or crawling. Her pupils barely responded to bright light. Mental development was at the idiot level." When this patient died at age 2½, the brain weighed 650 gm. The normal brain-weight for the same age in Japanese people is 960 gm.

In the second case, generalized convulsions developed at age eight months and continued thereafter. At age three years, seven months, this patient underwent examination at Kumamoto University. "She was helpless, poorly nourished, and underdeveloped, an idiot child with a head circumference of 42 cm," said the examiners. "Her weight was 7,500 gm. (16.5 pounds). She was unable to perform any purposeful movements . . ."

Although Dr. Löfroth had completed his study of methyl mercury in March, 1969, it was seven months later, in October, 1969, that the U.S. Embassy in Stockholm alerted Washington to the doctor's frightening message. State Department Airgram A-691, sent October 29, 1969, from Stockholm, attached a copy of Löfroth's study. The airgram was marked at the top:

To: Department of State
DEPARTMENT PLEASE PASS DEPT OF HEW

On the left-hand side was a series of printed departmental initials and hand-written numerals, showing how many copies of the airgram went to which departments. Seven copies went to the Department of Health, Education and Welfare (HEW). (The CIA received *16* copies.) But the seven copies sent to HEW stirred little action. Löfroth's message, as capsulized in Airgram A-691, was this:

a) Crops grown from seed treated with mercury can cause accumulation in the food chain leading to man, both when the crop is consumed directly and when it is consumed via animal products. (The U.S. Department of Agriculture, to whom this aspect of mercury should have been highly interesting, received 10 copies of Airgram A-691.)

b) Mercury can be methylated by biological systems. Commercial fishing has been banned in certain Swedish waters because of dangerous levels of methyl mercury in fish.

c) The human fetus concentrates mercury in itself from the mother's body. "The data presently available indicate that the human fetus might be visibly affected at a methyl mercury intake of the mother-to-be several times less than the intake affecting a non-pregnant adult," said Airgram A-691, quoting Löfroth.

Finally, those 175 federal officials who received a copy of Airgram A-691 learned that:

d) Mercury is known to cause serious genetic damage at very low levels of contamination.

It is to this, the most dangerous aspect of mercury poisoning, that we now turn.

District Health Officer George K. Fair, stationed at Las Cruces, New Mexico, reported to the New Mexico State Department of Health and Social Services on January 7, 1970, that three Alamogordo children had fallen ill with a disease of the central nervous system. Dr. Fair also reported that some of the family's hogs had died with "the blind staggers" three months earlier.

That afternoon, on a hunch, Medical Services Division Director Dr. Bruce Storrs said it sounded to him like heavy metal poisoning, arsenic or maybe mercury. Urine samples were dispatched east to the Food and Drug Administration's Toxicology Branch in Atlanta.

On January 11, both Amos and Dorothy Jean Huckleby entered the hospital in El Paso. Amos was deaf and blind. Dorothy Jean was raving.

FDA's Atlanta lab reported high levels of mercury in urine from the three Huckleby children.

6. Genetics:

The mutagens

Mercury's ability to cause genetic damage first came under suspicion at Minamata Bay. Physicians performing autopsies on Japanese children noted certain abnormalities that they could not attribute to direct mercury poisoning. It appeared as if the mercury eaten in fish at Minamata had entered the testes or ovaries of parents, damaged sex cells, and thus passed on genetic damage to the offspring. Severe mental and physical retardation—so-called mongolian idiocy (Down's syndrome) —resulted. The Mrak Commission had signaled the same warning, noting that

a particularly subtle danger from wide-scale use of pesticides lies in the possibility that some of them may be damaging to the hereditary material. If this is so, we may be unwittingly harming our descendants. Whether this is happening, and if so, what is the magnitude of the effect, is regrettably unknown.

Surely one of the greatest responsibilities of our generation is our temporary custody of the genetic heritage received from our ancestors. We must make every reasonable effort to insure that this heritage is passed on to future generations undamaged. To do less, we believe, is grossly irresponsible . . . The risk to future generations though difficult to assess in precise terms, is nevertheless very real. The prevention of any unnecessary mutational damage is one of our most important and immediate responsibilities. (pp. 568, 571).

The Mrak Report then says, "Some mercurials are known mutagens, presumably owing to their content of Hg [metallic mercury]." The report lists mercury pesticides (chiefly methyl mercury) as "compounds which by their structure may possibly affect DNA either directly or after enzymatic activation into reactive compounds. Among these are mercurials, some of which are known mutagens. . . ." (pp. 606, 608).

To understand the hazard of genetic damage by mercury we should look briefly at the human genetic mechanism. Human beings are made up of cells—some 50 trillion in a normal adult. The average human begins life, however, as a single cell, the fertilized ovum. Humans grow by the process of cell-division, called mitosis. During mitosis the cell divides itself into two identical cells. These in turn divide until we have four cells, then eight, then 16 and so on. Each cell carries inside it a complex set of instructions that determine how the cell will operate chemically, whether the cell will function as a part of a toenail or a brain, for example. The cell's instructions are contained in chromosomes. In human beings each cell contains 23 pairs of chromosomes.

Chromosomes contain the chemical blueprints according to which the human body constructs itself after the ovum is fertilized by a male sex cell at the moment of conception. Sex cells are produced in the gonads of adult humans. In the male, sperm cells are made in the testes; in females, egg cells are made in the ovaries. The production of sex cells involves a special cell-dividing process called meiosis. Meiosis is a cell division in which the chromosomes first group themselves into pairs and are then distributed to the newly created sex cells, *one* from each pair to each new cell. Thus meiosis produces sex cells, cells in which there are only half the number of chromosomes found in normal human cells. Human sex cells contain only 23 chromosomes, whereas normal human cells contain 23 *pairs* of chromosomes. When the 23 single chromosomes in sex cells seek partners to bring their number back to the full 46, a single cell is created, with 23 pairs of chromosomes, half from the mother, half from the father. Almost immediately the new single cell begins mitosis—dividing itself until it is two cells, then four, eight, 16, then a new human being.

Certain kinds of chemicals, called mutagens, have strange effects upon mitosis and meiosis. Mutagens enter into the chemical structure of cells and their chromosomes, causing chemical instructions to go haywire. Mercury is one such chemical mutagen.

Studies of mutagenicity originated in 1927 when Dr. Hermann J. Muller demonstrated that ionizing radiation caused inheritable damage in fruit flies *(Drosophila melanogaster)*. Between 1927 and 1945 many scientists suspected that certain chemicals could have the same genetic effects as radiation, but it wasn't until World War II that laboratory evidence proved chemical mutagenicity—specifically, mustard gas-damaged the sex cells of *Drosophila*. Since 1945 mutagenicity has increasingly come to scientific attention as a major public health hazard.

Whether a particular chemical damages human sex cells is difficult to determine. Direct experimentation on large human populations is obviously ruled out on moral grounds (though it might be said that some industrialists have been indirectly performing such experiments on populations world-wide in recent years). Instead of experimenting on humans directly, geneticists have developed laboratory experiments using plants and animals. Such species reproduce more rapidly and in greater number than humans, and their reproduction can be controlled so they make good vehicles for observing inherited changes. Two favorite species studied in genetic laboratories since World War II are the onion plant, *Allium cepa,* and the fly *Drosophilia*. But does information about genetic damage in onion roots and fruit flies tell us anything about potential genetic damage in humans? Answering this question, geneticist Theodosius Dobzhansky and author-scientist Isaac Asimov have written:

An important assumption in [genetic experiments on fruit flies] is that the machinery of inheritance and mutation is essentially the same in all creatures and that therefore knowledge gained from very simple species (even from bacteria) is applicable to man. *There is overwhelming evidence to indicate that this is true in general,* although there are specific instances where it is not completely true and scientists must tread softly while drawing conclusions. (Emphasis added.)

In December, 1967, Swedish geneticists Claes Ramel
and Jan Magnusson compiled results of two years' work.
They had studied the effects of mercury on plants and
animals, attempting to assess mercury's ability to produce genetic damage. Their reports (published in 1969)
stated that

> mercury compounds are extremely efficient in caus-
> ing disturbances of the mitotic [cell-dividing] appa-
> ratus, *resulting in changes in the normal chromo-
> some number* . . . Mercurials given in food to
> *Drosophila* larvae or adult flies obviously reach the
> gonads where they cause chromosome disturbances,
> presumably similar in nature as the ones observed
> cytologically in plant cells [*Allium cepa*]. (Empha-
> sis added.)

Ramel and Magnusson had fed *Allium* (the onion) , and
many generations of the fruit fly, *Drosophila,* food contaminated with mercury at various levels. The two investigators recognized the hazards of comparing human
reactions to reactions of flies and onions. Yet they noted
that mercury, and especially methyl mercury, is an extremely stable compound in mammals.

> Therefore [Ramel and Magnusson argue] there is
> reason to believe that, if these compounds reach the
> gonads, they do this in the same chemical form in
> humans as compared to *Drosophila*. In such a case
> the genetic effects can be expected to be similar.

Ramel and Magnusson's tests showed that methyl mercury is an extremely potent agent causing an aberration
in cell division called c-mitosis. In fact, by comparison
with the standard agent (a chemical called colchicine)
known to produce c-mitosis in *Allium,* Ramel judged

methyl mercury to be 1,000 times as potent an agent. In *Allium* roots, mercury's c-mitotic action caused changes in cells' meiotic systems, *giving rise to cells containing an abnormal number of chromosomes.*

In *Drosophila,* Ramel and Magnusson observed similar abnormalities in chromosome numbers and concluded that interference in the meiotic system, caused by mercury's c-mitotic agency, was responsible. Full c-mitosis in *Allium* begins at levels as low as 50 ppb and partial damage is observed at levels much lower.

These observations are of interest [argue Ramel and Magnusson] from a practical point of view in relation to the mercury pollution of the environment . . . This pollution includes some important human food stuff, like eggs and fresh water fishes, and therefore it obviously is of interest to establish what kind of human health risks may be involved. With reference to the experimental data, the genetic effects of such a health problem primarily concern the risk of an induction of cells with aberrant chromosome numbers. *This might cause an increase for instance of trisomic defects like mongolism or Klinefelter's syndrome.* (Emphasis added.)

Mongolism, as is well known, involves certain physical deformities and moderate-to-severe mental retardation. Klinefelter's syndrome is characterized by atrophied testes, the absence of living spermatozoa in the semen, and sometimes excessive development of male mammary glands. Both mongolism and Klinefelter's syndrome have been recognized since 1959 as resulting from an abnormal number of chromosomes.

Answering the question, "What kinds of effects on the human being do mutations produce?" the Mrak Report says:

Perhaps the most important fact to emphasize is that there is no single effect. Since every part of the body and every metabolic process is influenced by genes [which are part of the instruction mechanisms of chromosomes] to a greater or lesser extent, it comes as no surprise that the range of effects produced by gene alterations includes every kind of structure and process. (p. 569.)

The report continues:

. . . [T]he major statistical impact of a mutation increase on the human population would be to add the burden of mild mutational effects. This would make the population weaker, more prone to disease, and more likely to succumb to an effect that otherwise would be resisted. (p. 571)

All of this, of course, depends upon the amount of mercury poison reaching the gonads of adult human beings. Studies of this question in humans appear to be lacking, but it seems reasonable to assume that mercury carried in the blood stream will reach the gonads. In mice, it has been determined by careful laboratory measurement, mercury actually concentrates in the gonads. The same thing is known from lab experiments with trout.

As for the blood of human beings, it was announced in the *Archives of Environmental Health* in August, 1970, that three Swedish investigators noted "statistically significant" chromosome damage in red blood cells. The investigators' subjects had been eating mercury-contaminated fish about three times a week. If we figure servings of 150 grams each, a common assumption among mercury investigators, we find total consumption of one pound per week. The level of concentration of mercury in the fish was determined to run between 1,000 and 7,000 ppb—a level of contamination found in some fish in many of the surface waters of the United States today.

There remain other disturbing signs of danger from mercury. A June, 1970, literature-review by H. V. Malling, J. S. Wassom and S. S. Epstein, published in the *Newsletter of the Environmental Mutagen Society* (P.O. Box Y, Oak Ridge, Tenn. 37830; $10/yr.) raised the possibility that mercury can cause cancer:

> The carcinogenic [cancer-causing] potential of mercury or its products has not yet been thoroughly investigated. Early studies involving mercury, mercuric acetate, and mercuric chloride *show carcinogenic activity for mercury* and none for mercuric acetate and mercuric chloride. A recent publication has also suggested the possible role of mercury as an agent that enhances the activity of some carcinogens. (Emphasis added.)

Epstein is chief of Laboratories of Environmental Toxicology and Carcinogenesis, Children's Cancer Research Foundation, Boston. Malling directs the Environmental Mutagen Information Center headquartered at the AEC's Oak Ridge [Tenn.] National Laboratory, which is operated under contract by Union Carbide. Wassom assists Malling. In conclusion, Malling, Wassom and Epstein said:

> The genetic effects of mercury and its compounds have been illustrated in a number of papers [they

cite 13 of them, three by Claes Ramel as summarized elsewhere in this chapter]. The effects shown in these papers indicate a possible mutagenic effect of mercurials. Supporting evidence for these findings can be obtained by a review of papers concerned with the interaction of mercury compounds with nucleic acids and their constituents [they cite eight studies]. These genetic data have been derived from non-human systems but a Danish survey conducted in 1969 showed that Danes who had eaten large amounts of fish with high methyl mercury concentrations had significantly higher frequencies of lymphocyte chromosome aberrations than comparable controls.

None of the Danish fish eaters showed clinical symptoms of poisoning by mercury. Said the Mrak Report about findings like this:

Most, if not all, agents which induce inactivating DNA alterations or chromosome breaks *in vivo* have also been found to induce mutations, cancer, and teratogenic effects, when examined in the proper test system. (p. 605).

Still, officials in Washington continued to ignore the warnings.

In the OB ward at the Bernalillo County Medical Center in Albuquerque, Lois Huckleby waited to be wheeled to the delivery room to give birth to her sixth child. Two nurses in green caps and gowns were already making preparations for her there, laying out the instruments with rapid precision.

"I wonder," said the younger nurse, "what it will look like."

"Who knows?" said the other. "Maybe it'll be perfectly all right."

And so it seemed, for on March 22, 1970, Lois Huckleby gave birth to a fine-looking baby boy, whom the doctors pronounced perfectly healthy. And he was named after the archangel Michael, for gladness.

But when summer came to the southern New Mexico desert country, baby Michael cried a lot. A neighbor observed that perhaps it was simply because of the heat.

7. The Polluters:

Lot of talk, little action

During the weeks following December 8, 1969, when Ernestine Huckleby fell from the monkey bar at school and went home complaining of vague pains, the federal government continued to regard mercury hazards with detachment—at least until February 17, 1970, when NBC News spread the Huckleby story across the country.

Within 24 hours of the news broadcast, Dr. Harry Hays, then director of the Pesticide Regulation Division in the U.S. Department of Agriculture (USDA), announced the conclusion of "ten years" of research on the dangers of mercurial pesticides. He pronounced mercury "an imminent hazard," and said he was canceling registration (under the Federal Insecticide, Fungicide and Rodenticide Act of 1947) of 17 alkyl-mercury fungicides, chiefly the group known as "panogen." Further, he wired the major panogen supplier,

Nor-Am, the Chicago-based subsidiary of the Morton-Norwich chemical conglomerate, to recall its fungicide from dealers' shelves. On March 4, 1970, Agriculture Secretary Clifford Hardin announced cancellation of registration of methyl mercury products in addition to the panogen group.

Until that month, the American public knew little about the dangers of mercury—mainly a few fragmented details about the strange affliction of the Huckleby children. Then on March 20 Norvald Fimreite, a graduate student researcher at Western Ontario University, released to the press a letter he had sent the day before to Canadian Wildlife Service officials in which he described very high mercury levels—up to 7.09 ppm—in fish from a major commercial fishing area, Lake St. Clair. Four days later the Ontario government closed its side of the lake to commercial fishing; on April 7 the state of Michigan closed the American side. Soon Manitoba closed all or part of its principal lakes. Ultimately some 1,500 miles of fishing water in five Canadian provinces were closed. Then the state of Ohio not only closed its portion of Lake Erie to commercial fishing but also requested a federal investigation of mercury pollution in Ohio waters. Thus did the U.S. government finally become cognizant of water pollution by mercury.

For two months federal officials avoided pointed questions from the press about mercury poisoning. But *The Washington Post*'s Victor Cohn managed twice to learn from sources within the Food and Drug Administration (FDA) that its officials weren't sure about the so-called "safe" level of mercury it had established for food fish.

On June 18 Secretary of the Interior Walter Hickel announced a ban on the use of 16 pesticides, including mercury compounds, on 534 million acres of federally controlled lands. A month later, he made the most candid statement of any administration official during this pollution crisis. He announced that mercury pollution was "an intolerable threat to the health and safety of Americans." Unfortunately, Secretary Hickel at the time did not demonstrate the political muscle needed to remedy the situation.

On July 29 Senator Philip Hart (D-Mich.) convened hearings before his Subcommittee on Energy, Natural Resources, and the Environment (Committee on Commerce) , and asked some pointed questions about mercury. Assistant Secretary of the Interior Carl L. Klein, testifying on behalf of the administration, tried to explain that mercury pollution had crept up on the government unawares. He did describe poisonings in the felt-hat industry "in past centuries" (not mentioning U.S. studies as late as 1940 which showed that between 8 and 11 percent of all workers in the felt-cutting trade suffered signs of mercury poisoning) . And he cited other studies that showed poisoning of cinnabar miners—a continuing problem.

Klein also pointed out that federal officials had missed the danger because mercury use in the chlor-alkali industry doubled between 1965 and 1969. He did not mention, however, that even in 1965 a Bureau of Mines report had predicted such an increase.

Klein told how Secretary Hickel had ordered the Federal Water Quality Administration (FWQA) and the U.S. Geological Survey to undertake an "intensive, far-reaching, ever-continuing investigation" using "new techniques of discovery and detection so fine as to distinguish in the billionth parts . . . new techniques that have only recently become available as the state of the art has improved." Actually these refined techniques had been in wide use as long as five years before.

Meanwhile, various agencies in the Nixon administration were suddenly encountering a mercury specter.

The Bureau of Water Hygiene, a unit of the Department of Health, Education and Welfare, discovered that it had no idea how much mercury might be safe in drinking water. The bureau then adopted a standard set by the Soviet Union 10 years before. Worse still, the bureau found it had no technique for determining mercury levels as low as a few parts per billion. "We got caught with our standards down," says chief chemist Dr. Benjamin Pringle.

So, too, in a sense, did the USDA, whose attempt to ban mercury compounds from agricultural use almost fell apart under judicial scrutiny. Nor-Am, having agreed to stop the sale of panogen, balked at the USDA's demand that existing stocks of panogen be recalled from dealers' shelves, claiming that recall would create an insurmountable and hazardous hardship for the company. Later, a U.S. District Court in Chicago, at Nor-Am's request, enjoined the department from banning the methyl mercury pesticides. But then on November 9 U.S. Court of Appeals Judge Walter J. Cummings, holding that Nor-Am had not exhausted all remedies available under law and that it should have asked for an administrative hearing within the USDA before going to court, overthrew the opinion of the District Court and thereby upheld the USDA's ban.

The new U.S. Environmental Protection Agency,

which took over USDA's pesticide regulation authority in December, 1970, says it plans to enforce the ban on mercurials. Nor-Am, for its part, says it will go to the U.S. Supreme Court for the right to sell methyl mercury to farmers and seed dealers. At this writing, alkyl mercurials are still doing a brisk business in the United States.

Two days after Secretary Hickel acknowledged the dangers of mercury, the Justice Department announced it would take the biggest polluters to court for illegal dumping of mercury wastes into U.S. waters. Justice said it would invoke the 1899 Refuse Act, which empowers the Army Corps of Engineers to issue permits for the dumping of waste materials into navigable waterways and their tributaries, and provides penalties up to $2,500 per day for unlicensed dumping. (Under a provision of the law the judge may award all or part of the fine to the person who first takes such information to a U.S. attorney and requests legal action, even if the complainant ultimately initiates the court action himself.)

The eight companies named by the government suit were: Georgia-Pacific Corporation, plant at Bellingham, Washington; Olin Mathieson Chemical Corporation, Niagara Falls, New York, and Augusta, Georgia; Oxford Paper Company, Rumford, Maine; Weyerhaeuser Company, Longview, Washington; Diamond Shamrock Corporation, Delaware City, Delaware, and Muscle Shoals, Alabama; Allied Chemical Company, Solvay, New York; International Mining and Chemical Company, Orrington, Maine, and Pennwalt Chemical Company, Calvert City, Kentucky.

Later, under prodding from Ralph Nader, the Interior Department announced the names of the nation's 50 major mercury polluters, which resembled a blue-chip catalogue: Wyandotte Chemical, Dow Chemical, Tenneco Chemical, Allied Chemical, Detrex Chemical, Diamond Shamrock, Georgia-Pacific, Olin Mathieson, Oxford Paper, Weyerhaeuser, B. F. Goodrich Chemical, Pennwalt Chemical, General Aniline and Film, Stauffer Chemical, PPG Industries, Riegel Paper, Westinghouse, Aluminum Company of America, Monochem Incorporated, Hooker Electro-Chemical, Woodbridge Chemical, Monsanto Chemical, General Electric.

Simultaneously, Secretary Hickel reported a nationwide reduction in industrial mercury discharges, from 287 pounds to 40 pounds per day. The figures appear questionable, inasmuch as the U.S. Bureau of Mines and the U.S. Geological Survey both estimate that since 1930 mercury losses into the American environment have averaged one million pounds per year. Therefore, the average mercury pollution *per day* for the past 40 years has been 2,739 pounds, or almost 10 times the higher discharge cited by Secretary Hickel.

The first company taken to court by the Department of Justice was the Olin Corporation. But this action ended when the department accepted a promise from Olin that it would cut its pollution of the Niagara River to one-half pound of mercury per day, after which it would submit further plans for reduction.

Not one of the accused companies paid a cent in fines, nor did any corporate executive risk jail for polluting.

The only citizen-based legal action against mercury polluters has fizzled. The Bass Anglers Sportsman So-

ciety of America, Inc., with headquarters in Mont-
gomery, Alabama, on July 22, 1970 filed suit under the
1899 Refuse Act, naming 216 Alabama companies, the
Secretary of the Army, and the Alabama Water Improve-
ment Commission as defendants.

Federal judges in Texas and Alabama ruled the Bass
Anglers have no standing to bring action against anyone.
Since mercury pollution is a *criminal* matter, these judges
ruled, the state (meaning the U.S. Attorney in Alabama) must prosecute.

The Bass Anglers are appealing. Meantime, since two
federal courts have said that the state must bring charges
if anything is to be done, what is the U.S. Attorney in
Alabama planning? Nothing at all. He wanted to, he
explained to Bass Anglers, but he says he queried the
U.S. Justice Department and received by return wire
this message: "Do not prosecute."

As if to epitomize the government's response to the
mercury crisis, when Sen. Winston Prouty (R-Vt.) on
July 30, 1970, called upon President Nixon to designate
mercury pollution an "imminent hazard" and thus gear
up federal control action more aggressively, the president
refused.

That autumn Lois and Ernest Huckleby heard from state health officials that their other son, Amos, and the two afflicted girls were making progress, learning to sit up by themselves again, learning to hold a spoon again.

But still baby Michael cried a lot.

8. The Workers:

"I'll send you a wreath."

Industrial fatalities caused by mercury poisoning have occurred since man first fractured the earth to mine quicksilver from cinnabar. In the United States in recent years, the number of victims has fluctuated between three and 11 annually. Nonfatal sicknesses caused by industrial poisoning remain largely unreported. Except in the manufacture of pesticides, workers today generally encounter only metallic and inorganic mercury on the job—poisonous and dangerous, but not to the extreme toxic extent of the organic alkyl mercurials.

Industrial poisoning by inorganc mercurials first occurred in America about 1865, when fur and felt workers reported having "the Danbury Shakes"—a fine, rhythmic tremor of the hands that soon spreads to the entire body if the victim continues working around mercury. When Danbury, Connecticut, was the center of the U.S. felt-hat manufacturing trade, "Shakes" afflicted workers who used mercuric nitrate as a "carroting agent" to improve the felting qualities of fur. The felt industry stopped relying on mercury in the late 1950s. But the Danbury Shakes now afflict workers in other industries.

The symptoms of mercury poisoning aren't the same in all cases. Workers who receive a small dose of mercury each day develop symptoms of chronic poisoning. Workers who accidentally ingest large amounts of mercury at one time develop symptoms of acute poisoning. *Chronic poisoning* leads to disintegration of the nervous system, and occasionally to kidney damage resembling nephritis. *Acute poisoning* leads to vomiting, abdominal pain, sometimes bloody diarrhea, then severe kidney injury, perhaps central nervous system damage, then death.

Workers who come down with chronic low-level poisoning symptoms frequently are unaware of what has hit them. The early symptoms are nonspecific: fatigue, nervous anxiety, insomnia, impairment of memory, loss of appetite, perhaps headaches. Over the long run, low-level central nervous system damage will begin to develop, the characteristic tremor in fingertips or eyelids or tongue, sores in the mouth, difficulty urinating, tightness and pains in the chest, coughing, difficulty breathing, and erethrism, a peculiar anti-social reaction.

Erethrism has been best described by the British specialist in occupational diseases, Dr. P. Lesley Bidstrup, in her authoritative *Toxicity of Mercury and its Compounds:*

> This is the most difficult manifestation of chronic mercury poisoning to assess, particularly when tremor is absent and the patient is unknown to the

doctor making the examination. Nervousness, irritability, a tendency to blush easily, and a history —often best obtained from friends or members of the family—of change of temperament, a tendency to avoid meeting friends and unexplained outbursts of temper, should cause the physician or psychiatrist to enquire carefully into the possibility of exposure to mercury as a cause of the symptoms before attributing them to anxiety or 'neurasthenia.'

Erethrism used to afflict felt-hat workers, making them "mad as a hatter."

By far the highest incidence of industrial mercury poisonings results from inhalation of elemental mercury vapor. In Great Britain between 1956 and 1960, 19 of the 22 reported industrial mercury poisonings involved mercury vapors. [In England, mercurialism has been a reportable disease—one that physicians *must* report to health authorities whenever they encounter its symptoms—since 1899. Yet mercurialism, or chronic mercury poisoning, is still not a reportable disease in America.]

Mercury vapors abound in certain U.S. workplaces. When Ralph Nader testified before Sen. Philip Hart's subcommittee July 29, 1970, he placed into the record a portion of a job description published by the Windsor Locks, Connecticut, plant of Hamilton Standard, a division of United Aircraft. The job title, said Nader, was "Maintenance mechanic, mechanical," and the company's own description of "working conditions" included the following: "Frequent exposure to grease, oil, gases, *mercury vapors,* dirt, dust, inclement weather make job somewhat disagreeable." (Emphasis added.)

Nader read into the record other descriptions of American and Canadian workplaces. They were originally supplied to Anthony Mazzocchi of the Oil, Chemical and Atomic Workers' Union (OCAW) by workers speaking up at public meetings. OCAW has published five volumes of verbatim testimony taken at public meetings around the nation.

A worker at Dow Chemical's Sarnia, Canada, plant (the Canadian-managed, American-owned plant that is being sued by the state of Ohio for polluting Lake Erie), told a public meeting:

> We all know there is a terrific health hazard with mercury. It's become a common thing to see it lay around on the floor and on the ground. The window cleaners come in and clean windows in our unit, and half an hour after they start to do their job, their squeegees become so covered with silver that they can't use them any longer, and the buckets become tainted because of the mercury they scrape off the windows.

An employee of Woodbridge Chemical Company in Hawthorne, New Jersey, reported:

> Most of our products are mercury . . . When we pack it, the dust from this here powder gets into our lungs, even though we have a mask on. And they're supposed to have a blower. But every time the doctor comes in to test me for the mercury that I inhale from this powder, they always tell me they should take me down to the still [mercury distilling unit] instead of sending scrap mercury, because I have more mercury in my system than we collect in the scrap container. We have so much mercury, I'm telling you, the mercury. They put 25

flasks [weighing 76 pounds apiece] and they say, "Dump them." They see you dump 25. They bring 50 more. And how much of this mercury am I inhaling? I told my foreman, "You know, I'm going to be in the cemetery." He said, "Well, I tell you, I'll send you a wreath." He said it as a joke. But he was serious.

Workers in many occupations today endure unnecessary mercury hazards. Cinnabar mining "exposes the worker to a definite risk," says Dr. M. C. Battigelli, a professor at the University of Pittsburgh Graduate School of Public Health. But a still "greater risk is associated with subsequent operations at the refining plant, particularly in connection with cleansing of the distillation columns," adds Dr. Battigelli.

One mining operation caught fire in 1803 and some 900 people living in the vicinity came down with mercury poisoning, apparently from the vapors. This was at the large Idria mine in Yugoslavia. In recent years, serious poisoning of quicksilver miners has been reported in the Peruvian Andes, on the Philippine Islands and in California.

Other industrial poisonings have occurred in the manufacture of dry cell batteries, the repairing of direct-current electrical meters, the brewing of beer (where mercury plugs allow gases to escape from huge vats during fermentation) and the gilding of buttons for military costumes. Industrial poisonings occur regularly, if infrequently, in nearly all of the industries listed in the Appendix, Industrial Uses of Mercury.

Poisoning of laboratory workers seems to be occurring with increasing frequency. Industrial hygienist Dr. Leonard J. Goldwater has reported clinical evidence of chronic mercury poisoning among workers in one university laboratory. Dr. Neville Grant, the Washington University physician, points to a study of 47 Pennsylvania hospital laboratories: excessive mercury vapors existed in six locations (12.7 percent).

Laboratory workers need to be especially careful in handling mercury because, when dropped, the metal splatters into thousands of tiny beads and slips easily into cracks. There it rapidly vaporizes, spreading dangerous poison throughout the ambient air. Dr. Goldwater has pointed out that a ball of mercury with a one-inch diameter has a surface area of 3.1 square inches. However, broken into droplets measuring 1/32 of an inch in diameter, the same amount of mercury presents a surface area of approximately 100 square inches. Mercury dropped on laboratory floors is thus quite accessible to the atmosphere.

There is historical evidence that the famous French mathematician Blaise Pascal and the British electrical researcher Michael Faraday both suffered from chronic mercurialism resulting from laboratory exposure.

One highly dangerous practice is to tap the end of a cigarette on a lab bench contaminated by miniscule droplets of mercury. The heat of the cigarette will vaporize the mercury instantly, delivering the full dose directly into the lungs.

The American Conference of Governmental Industrial Hygienists has recommended numerical standards for ambient air levels of mercury. The recommended standard for inorganic mercury and mercury vapors is 0.1 milligrams per cubic meter of air. This is called a MAC value—Maximum Allowable Concentration value. Such a MAC value for mercury in the air would allow a

normal worker to absorb through his lungs some 500
micrograms of mercury per day. The human body, however, is thought by some scientists to be able to tolerate
daily doses of only 175 to 350 micrograms per day. But
500 micrograms per day, they fear, might bring on poisoning symptoms in some workers. (See Appendix,
Workplace Standards.)

Television reporters were waiting in Alamogordo when Lois Huckleby returned that day from Albuquerque, where specialists had just examined baby Michael, now eight months old. Lois Huckleby looked squarely at the newsmen and, even before they could ask, said:

"The baby is blind."

9. The FDA:

How safe is "safe?"

On September 17, 1970, the Food and Drug Administration announced that people who rub hand or skin lotion over large areas of their bodies every day risk "an appreciable hazard of poisoning." The hazard, it said, comes from the mercury that is added to the lotions to kill germs.

In an interview with the Associated Press, Dr. Alfred Weissler, chief of the FDA's cosmetics section, explained that FDA has no legislative authority to compel removal of potentially dangerous mercury from cosmetics. FDA, it seems, relies on the $6 billion-per-year cosmetics industry to regulate itself. (An FDA study in 1969 revealed 20 percent of 159 drug and cosmetic preparations intended for skin use contained bacterial contamination; in more than half the cases the offending germ was classified as a possible infection agent—

which gives one some notion of the past effectiveness of self-regulation by the cosmetics industry.)

According to the AP dispatch, officials of the Toilet Goods Association said that mercury is used in four of 18 product classifications—creams, lotions, hair preparations and facial makeup. FDA officials added that they believed some 40 cosmetic products on the market contain the poison. The FDA declined to identify the products by name.

The FDA lacks the authority to force recall of lotions it admits may be poisoning a lot of well-tanned Americans who may not happen to read FDA announcements in the *Federal Register* or the back pages of *The Washington Post*. But it is empowered to regulate the marketing of food and drug products. Thus the FDA emerged as the great protector of the public's good health when it pounced on 25,000 vitamin pills made from seal livers and marketed through an obscure health food store. FDA seized the vitamin pills off the shelf and promptly trumpeted its action to the press-at-large. Meanwhile, except through some of the nation's larger newspapers that happened to carry the AP's skin lotion story, no official notice had gone out to American families that their favorite soothing skin preparation, used daily, might be affecting their nerves or the lives of their unborn children.

In October 1970—full seven months after Norvald Fimreite revealed mercury pollution throughout the Great Lakes region—the FDA finally got around to checking the mercury content of the American diet. By this time mercury had been discovered in fresh-water fish in 33 states at levels called "unsafe" by FDA.

The FDA's safety level, however, is vague. It specifies that no product shall be deemed "safe" if it contains more than 0.5 parts per million of mercury. That is, if you had a million pounds of the substance—whatever it may be, from wheat to carrots to fish flesh—and if you refined it chemically so as to remove the mercury, you'd extract no more than half a pound of mercury from the million edible pounds with which you began. That's a concentration of 0.5 ppm, and it's the FDA's safety standard for all food fish.

The FDA set this standard in a hurry in July, 1969, right after *Environment* magazine reported that mercury was becoming ubiquitous. Or, rather, the agency set *part* of a standard. Actually, FDA officials call the standard a "guideline," but the guideline only specifies a concentration that is prohibited: anything over 0.5 ppm. The FDA standard doesn't say *how much* one ought or ought not to eat of foods contaminated at "safe" levels.

Thus, to give a practical example of the way the FDA's regulation is being interpreted, the state health department in New Mexico has announced that certain fishing waters are "safe" because the fish in them are only polluted up to a level of 0.4 ppm. But it is plain that the poor fisherman who eats *two* "safe" pounds of fish from "safe" waters will ingest more total mercury than another fisherman who eats one pound of fish from the "contaminated" (0.5 ppm) waters of other lakes in New Mexico.

The FDA's concentration guideline (0.5 ppm) means nothing until it is linked to some specific amount of edible substance. Indeed, prohibiting a particular concentration, in this case anything over 0.5 ppm, may result in misleading appraisals of the mercury problem by the American people. It is the human body's total intake of mercury, and the particular mercury compound (s) involved, that determine the danger or safety of a person's diet, not the concentration of the mercury in the edible material.

The FDA's 1970 tests included 34 samples of each of 10 foodstuffs: flour, nonfat dry milk, sugar, potatoes, raw ground beef, chicken breast, shrimp, beef liver, hens' eggs and fluid whole milk. Note the omission of fin fish. By the end of the year, results on the first six foodstuffs revealed *no* mercury in *any* of the samples, not even trace levels, according to Caesar Roy in the FDA office of compliance.

In view of the findings reported after a similar survey of the Canadian diet by University of Toronto chemist Robert Jervis, the FDA's results appear highly questionable. Jervis and co-workers spent seven months performing some 300 activation analyses on biological samples taken from around the world, but mainly in Canada. In 21 samples of wheat taken from the United States, France and Japan, Jervis found levels averaging from 0.02 to 0.085 ppm mercury (except 0.15 ppm for Japan and 0.25 ppm for France). Jervis's findings have recently been questioned—they may be high by a factor of 10, it seems. Still, Jervis cites a 1969 study, reported in a journal published for activation analysts, of tests performed on American beef and pork. They averaged 0.1 ppm. Jervis also tested marine fish and concluded that tuna, among others, didn't show evidence of pollution. Marine fish averaged 0.01 to 0.08 ppm—a figure

considerably lower than the background level for fresh-
water fish, 0.2 ppm.

Jervis reported that human hair usually reflects the
presence of mercury in the body. Levels of 150 ppm in
human hair will occur at about the same time poisoning
symptoms occur, "depending on the individual's tolerance," said Jervis, without specifying a particular mercury compound. Jervis sampled the hair of Canadians
and concluded that the normal environmental level of
mercury in Canada now leaves concentrations in human hair that are below the poisoning level by a factor
of 10 to 20. Jervis concluded: "This is not considered
an adequate margin of safety by most toxicologists today, bearing in mind the differences in tolerance
thresholds among the population."

Moreover, Jervis cited a 1963 World Health Organization (WHO) standard for mercury concentrations in
food intended for human consumption. The standard is
0.05 ppm—10 times stricter than Canadian and FDA
health authorities have established as "safe." Said Jervis: "More than half of the foods analyzed had mercury
concentrations greater than the WHO 'suggested' MAC
[maximum allowable concentration]." Despite these
findings in Canada, FDA said as recently as January
1971 that it could find *no mercury whatever* in the
American diet.

According to at least two independent American scientists, the FDA's results are probably wide of the
mark. Dr. David Wilson at Vanderbilt University and
Dr. Thomas Clarkson at Rochester University suggest
that the FDA, through acid digestion of the biological
materials being sampled, may well have lost a lot of the
mercury. Volatilizing mercury—turning it into a vapor

—is difficult to avoid, says Victor Lambou of the Federal Water Quality Administration (FWQA) —now a division of the Environmental Protection Agency. In fact, many of the 1970 water and fish samples taken by FWQA appeared to contain less mercury than they probably contained because of the volatilization problem. Much of the 1970 work has to be repeated.

On October 30, 1970, Richard Ronk, mercury project officer in FDA's office of compliance, reported that several states in the West had already warned pregnant women to avoid eating fish from contaminated areas. "I think this is a good idea," said Ronk, "because we don't know how much mercury is a hazard to a fetus." Ronk's office has since reaffirmed this position. But the FDA has apparently made no great effort to publicize this important public health opinion.

In the wake of Ronk's warning came word from the Federal Trade Commission that Dr. West's "germ fighter" toothbrushes were treated with mercury and could "ultimately be dangerous to the consumer." The FTC also accused the manufacturer, Chemway Corporation, Wayne, New Jersey, of deceptive advertising when the company claimed that the "germ fighter" toothbrush kills germs likely to cause infectious mouth disease. At the same time, Professor Bruce McDuffie of the State University of New York at Binghamton reported finding mercury in canned tuna fish at levels up to 0.86 ppm. Despite their widespread six-month search for mercury in the New York environment, health officials once again appeared to be caught short by an independent researcher.

Professor McDuffie's announcement sent the FDA into a frenzy of tuna fish testing. Then FDA Commissioner Charles C. Edwards announced he was ordering one million cans of tuna fish off supermarket shelves. But at the same time he took the tuna off the shelves, Commissioner Edwards also announced that the tuna was "absolutely" safe to eat anyway. After 138 samples averaged 0.37 ppm mercury, with the highest being 1.12 ppm, FDA calculated that 23 percent of the 900 million cans of tuna processed in 1970 actually contained levels of mercury above the officially allowed 0.5 ppm. By mid-March 1971, tuna testing revealed only 3.6 percent of the cans contaminated. The remainder was adjudged "safe."

Yet many people could not forget that Commissioner Edwards had stressed in his original announcement that the contaminated tuna fish he had ordered off grocers' shelves was really "absolutely" safe to eat. "The guideline [0.5 ppm] offers a substantial margin for safety," Commissioner Edwards had said.

Dr. Les Ramsey, FDA's man on the Interagency Coordinating Committee on Mercury and Heavy Metals, says the FDA mercury standard contains a safety factor of 10. However, Dr. Ramsey admits that the normal standard for food additives and for chemicals (such as pesticides) artificially introduced into the environment contains a *normal* safety factor of 100. "For most of the food additives and pesticides on the market we try to keep a safety factor well *over* 100," says Dr. Ramsey, "and we usually succeed."

But in the case of mercury, setting a maximum allowable concentration value much tighter than 0.5 ppm would approach the background level for fresh-water fish, which seems to be 0.2 ppm or less. If the safety standard were set at background level and enforced, that would spell the end of fishing in America. Thus we find health officials rushing to set numerical standards based on skimpy evidence, under heavy pressure from economic forces which dwarf the demands of mere human health. Sportfishing in America is a billion-dollar industry.

Unfortunately, Commissioner Edwards's ambivalence over the toxicity of mercury colored much press coverage of the tuna fish contamination alarm. *Newsweek,* for example, made light of the whole thing this way:

> One part per million is not much; using that formula, a bartender could stretch a single ounce of vermouth over almost 500,000 superdry martinis. While health officials do not know how much mercury a human can safely ingest, the U.S. has adopted a very cautious standard of 0.5 ppm in food. . .

Against any likelihood that thousands of fish-eating Americans might come down with the gross symptoms of mercury poisoning, the FDA standard is perhaps "very cautious" and tuna fish is perhaps "absolutely" safe to eat once a week or so.

But from the viewpoint of birth defects, of cancer, of chromosomal aberrations, the FDA standard is anything but "very cautious." At least two widely respected Swedish investigators declare the U.S. standard to be twice as lax as it ought to be. And by World Health Organization figures our FDA standard is not "very cautious." It is loose and permissive. Recommendations of the United Nations' Food and Agriculture Organization Working Party and the WHO Expert Committee on Pesticide Residues regarding mercury read as follows:

Level causing no toxicological effect in rats: A no-effect level has not been demonstrated. *Estimate of acceptable daily intake for man:* The level of 0.1 ppm, equivalent to 0.005 mg/kg [milligrams per kilogram] body-weight per day, produced a slight effect in the rat. Even if this figure were to be adopted as a maximum no-effect level and the customary safety factor applied, this would give an acceptable daily intake for man of 0.00005 mg/kg body-weight. This is tantamount to zero. *It is undesirable that for the general population there should be any increase in the natural intake of mercury.* (Emphasis added.)

On Christmas Eve, 1970, the news carried reports that 89 percent of all the swordfish on sale in the United States may contain mercury levels above the permissible 0.5 ppm. These figures have since been confirmed. Swordfish tests showed 62 samples of frozen whole steaks, filets and chunks contained an average of 0.93 ppm, with the range running from 0.18 (background level) up to 2.4 ppm, which is very serious contamination. Still, FDA officials announced "there is no cause for alarm." FDA Deputy Commissioner James Grant did say, however, that "regular consumption" of swordfish would be an "unnecessary and avoidable risk."

It should be noted that FDA sentries had already checked both tuna and swordfish for mercury dangers, failing to turn up any almost certainly because of defective sampling technique or analytic method.

FDA's representative on the special federal Interagency Coordinating Committee on Mercury and Heavy Metals, Dr. Les Ramsey, explains that the FDA's recommended maximum allowable concentration for food (0.5 ppm) is based on the "latest, best" evidence. We asked Dr. Ramsey if mutagenicity had been taken into consideration in setting the FDA standard.

"Mercury hasn't been earmarked as a mutagen," he said.

Who in FDA would know about mercury's mutagenicity?

"Marvin Legator," said Dr. Ramsey.

Dr. Marvin Legator is chief of the cell biology branch, Bureau of Science, in FDA. Legator served as executive secretary of the Advisory Panel on Mutagenicity, advising the Mrak Commission.

"We haven't looked at the mutagenicity of mercury in our FDA labs," says Dr. Legator. "I'd suggest Heinrich Malling at Oak Ridge. He'd know about mercury."

In the meantime you are assured by FDA Commissioner Charles C. Edwards, M.D., that the mercury in your diet can't harm you a bit. But what about the children?

And the children's children?

(P.S. At presstime: On May 6, 1971, the F.D.A.—and Charles C. Edward—re-considered to a degree. The F.D.A. advised Americans to *stop* eating swordfish. Nine of ten samples tested contained excessive mercury.)

Amos came home for Christmas 1970 in his wheelchair, wearing dark glasses. With help now, he can take a step or two. His sister, Dorothy Jean—though a sample from her hair showed the highest level of mercury ever recorded in a human being—is doing much better. On crutches, she can walk 100 feet in 10 minutes.

Ernestine remains seriously afflicted at Gerald Champion Memorial Hospital in Alamogordo. Still blind and unable to speak, she manages a smile for special visitors. She plays with simple toys in her bed.

Then, there is Michael, no more than a fetus in his mother's womb when poisonous panogen spilled from the rat-gnawed sacks at Texico. Michael, named for gladness, is still blind, too.

10. Questions and Answers

The mercury crisis has produced many public health questions but almost no reassuring answers.

To begin at the level of cell biology, scientists do not yet know exactly how mercury damages nerve cells, fibers and synapses. Until these mechanisms are illuminated by laboratory research, antidotes for mercury poisoning will remain unavailable. The genetic effects of mercury, its ability to produce birth defects, and its cancer-producing qualities all need description and elaboration. Much work remains to be done identifying the action of various mercury compounds as they move through air and water environments to enter food chains. The effects of mercury compounds on water organisms, on bacteria, plants, insects and animals need elucidation.

Mercury pollution has not stopped by any means.

And the mercury that has been dumped into U.S. waterways during the last 70 years remains there, methylating slowly, percolating outward into the earth's biosphere. Somewhere between 165 and 181 million pounds of mercury have passed through American industrial establishments since 1900, and most of it has come out in some new form. Where all this mercury now resides is a question that must be answered.

Most urgent, research must be initiated to establish standardized procedures for monitoring the environment for mercury pollution. Although some work remains to be done perfecting inexpensive, reliable, portable instruments that can measure mercury, much more work is required to develop better sampling techniques. Mercury gets lost very easily and *any* loss is significant when one is looking for nanogram levels of contamination (a nanogram is one billionth of a gram).

Meanwhile, many Americans will be asking themselves some hard questions. Thousands, in fact, already are wondering whether it is safe to eat fish. But, once again, reliable answers aren't available. Lacking them, one should probably avoid swordfish. A normal serving of swordfish—say 150 grams—may well contain too much mercury. As a matter of fact, all fish concentrate mercury in their flesh, so whether you eat swordfish, tuna or trout you are getting more mercury than you would if you took your protein other ways. Other foods contain mercury as well, but not at levels near those in fish. It would probably be best to wait for a year or two, until more is known about the low-level effects of mercury on humans, before resuming a daily (or even once-weekly) diet of fish. It is now known to scientists the alkyl mercury compounds found in fish can destroy brain cells if they are ingested in quantities measured as micrograms. Genetic damage may occur at much lower levels. The authors believe that *pregnant women should avoid eating any fish*.

Some Americans are asking if water supplies have been contaminated by mercury. The uncertain answer is: Apparently not yet. Having surveyed 142 municipal water supply systems in 13 states by mid-December 1970, the U.S. Bureau of Water Hygiene reported finding mercury in concentrations above 1.0 ppb in only three water supplies. None was higher than 2.6 ppb, though raw water samples from some portions of the nation's great waterways—the Mississippi and Rio Grande rivers, for example—contained concentrations as high as 8 ppb near industrial sources of mercury pollution. Raw water concentrations were measured after removal of suspended sediment. Suspended sediment is known to contain mercury concentrations above water-background levels by a factor of from five to 25.

HEW's Bureau of Water Hygiene in May 1970 set a "tentative" standard for drinking water: 0.005 ppm (5 ppb). The bureau apparently doesn't know whether this is a safe level or not, but it *thinks* it is.

One thing is certain: Once the federal government sets its official standard for drinking water, no one will call for a raw-river-water standard or an industrial effluent standard to be set *more stringent* than the drinking water standard. But the facts of the case may require just that. Microscopic water plants such as phytoplankton may be more sensitive to mercury than people are, and life's food chain begins with the water plants. Our health depends on their health.

Three Florida researchers, Harriss, White and Mcfarlane, recently concluded in *Science:*

> It is clear that concentrations of mercurial com-
> pounds well below the proposed water-quality
> standards [5 ppb] can have detrimental effects on
> phytoplankton. . .The long-term effects of mercu-
> ry pollution below concentration of 1 ppb must be
> determined to establish adequate water-quality
> standards.

The three Florida scientists also said:

> We conclude that the use of organomercurial com-
> pounds in any way that permits their discharge
> into natural waters should be stopped as soon as
> possible.

So we have another unanswered question: How soon is possible? That, of course, is a political question.

Then there are those questions inspired by the de-bunkers of danger. For example, they say volcanoes have always added mercury to the environment; so why blame the pollution on industrial wastes? True, volcanoes have added large quantities of mercury to the environment—the seas alone are now estimated to contain 500 metric tons of mercury. It may also be true that swordfish and tuna absorb their mercury from natural "leaks" where sea water or the local small-fish population contain elevated levels. It seems unlikely—but it may prove to be so. (In the meantime, natural source or not, the methyl mercury in ocean fish is still a deadly poison to be wary of.) It is even more unlikely that fresh-water fish get their mercury from natural depos-its, except in a few very rare locations. Sufficient stud-

ies have now been completed to say with reasonable
certainty that elevated levels of mercury in fresh-water
fish can almost invariably be traced to industrial
sources.

It has also been reported—by New York officials—
that mercury is measurable in preserved fish at least 40
years old. Does that mean mercury pollution has always
been with us, that it's natural?

Henry L. Diamond, New York State's Environmental
Conservation Commissioner, announced finding excessive mercury in 12 preserved fish caught as long ago
as 1930. Diamond reported finding up to 1.03 ppm mercury in one blue pike caught in Irondequoit Bay, an
arm of Lake Ontario near Rochester, in 1939. Fish tak-
en from isolated waters—for example, smallmouth bass
from Long Pond and Boyd Pond deep in the Adirondacks in 1930—revealed levels of mercury exceeding
the FDA's guideline, 0.5 ppm.

But a dozen fish is an extremely small sample. Moreover, it is quite possible that these areas were polluted as
early as 1930 (or even as early as 1900) by the burning
of fossil fuels. Both coal and crude oil contain mercury;
burning them releases mercury vapor to the atmosphere. Part of the mercury may well have fallen out in
the Adirondacks.

Another question: Can mercury pollution be cleaned
out of our lakes and rivers?

The answer seems to be that no one has any clear
idea how to clean up the mercury fallout. Numerous
schemes have been proposed. Few have been tested.
Some of the advantages and disadvantages of various
methods are shown in the following chart:

Method	Advantages	Disadvantages	Unknowns
Dredging	Removes mercury entirely; possibility of mercury recovery	Disposal of dredged material; the process itself can perhaps release a large pulse of mercury; requires elaborate equipment	Ancillary ecological effects; cost
Covering with inactive clay or mercury-binding particulates (e.g., freshly ground quartz, feldspar, etc.)	Simplicity	May not be effective (lake turnover, erosion, reversible binding, etc.); mercury pulse	Cost; effectiveness
Covering with iron pyrite and clay overburden	Simplicity; works to put mercury in a more chemically inactive state; physically covers mercury sediments	Same as for clay and particulates; introduction of iron into lake	Ancillary ecological effects; cost
Reacting with H_2S to convert mercury to HgS	Works to put mercury in chemically inactive state	Difficulty to control action of this powerful reagent; difficult to direct the H_2S directly to the right physical spot; the resulting HgS is not physically covered	Ancillary ecological effects; cost; reaction time

Method	Advantages	Disadvantages	Unknowns
Raise pH of water	Might use lime which would tend to cover mercury deposits	Might cause air pollution; could spread mercury over wider area by releasing mercury from sediments	Ancillary ecological effects; cost
Plastic coatings	Simplicity; avoids lake turnover or sediment migration problems	Permanence?	Ancillary ecological effects; cost
Amalgamation with aluminum or other active metal	Simplicity	Puts another metal in the lake	Ancillary ecological effects; cost; effectiveness
Biological mining (e.g., with clams)	Minimum effect on ecology	Could increase the speed of methylmercury conversion; might not be possible for some streams	Cost; rate of mining; effectiveness

Courtesy: U.S. Atomic Energy Commission.

The ultimate question is: What can be done to prevent mercury pollution in the future?

First, congressional investigation of the public health and environmental protection communities should be reopened. We must examine the roles of various agencies and personnel. The mercury situation reveals that many public health officials come to their jobs unable—or unwilling—to search aggressively for health dangers in the environment, to analyze those dangers and then act upon that analysis.

Congressional investigators need particularly to look at the philosophical underpinnings of public health education. Why do public health personnel not emerge from their formal training vigilant, suspicious, armed with the latest techniques of discovery and analysis, unafraid to investigate all clues of environmental danger, knowledgeable in the means of publicizing their findings? As corporate technology widens and deepens its impact on our environment, citizens become increasingly dependent upon public health officials to protect them against odorless, tasteless poisons. Neglecting fundamental reform in public health education now could cost the nation very heavily in the near future.

In addition, we need much better data on how mercury and other dangerous metals are being used in America and throughout the world, and especially where they are being dumped. We may well need an accountability system for mercury (and other persistent, toxic substances) similar to the Atomic Energy Commission's system for keeping track of fissionable materials.

In 1968, the International Biological Program appointed Swedish ecologist Bengt Lundholm leader of a three-man team to study the feasibility of a global pollution monitoring network. Dr. W. Frank Blair at University of Texas and Dr. N. N. Smirnov of the Soviet Union served with Lundholm. Their mission: To organize scientific committees in their home nations and make recommendations two years hence.

In mid-February, 1970, the committee reported such a global monitoring system not only feasible but "necessary" because "a global crisis exists with respect to environmental quality." The committee urged immediate IBP action. The hope is to get a 20- to 40-station monitoring system started by 1972, the year the U.N. plans to hold a Conference on the Human Environment.

Clearly, what is needed most is a new style of citizen participation in the regulatory process. The development of counterpressures inside bureaucracies (corporate as well as governmental) must be studied. Ralph Nader has led the way in this direction. Now, more citizens must arm themselves with a new weapon—up-to-date information. And we must have more groups like the Barry Commoner-inspired Scientists' Institute for Public Information (SIPI) to meet the corporate "experts" on their own turf and to alert the public to impending dangers.

Basic reform legislation to implement new citizen access to the decision-making process, coupled with a scientific information effort on a grand scale, could turn the battle (which humanity is, for the present, losing) against environmental disaster. Senators Philip Hart (D.-Mich.) and George McGovern (D.-S.D.) and Congressman Morris Udall (D.-Ariz.) have introduced an Environmental Protection Act which would (a) grant all citizens a federally guaranteed right to a pollution-free environment; (b) open state and federal courts to antipollution suits by citizens; (c) give citizens standing before administrative agencies (to present the environmentalists' side of things); and (d) give citizens standing in state and federal agencies that are lax in enforcing antipollution standards.

Finally, the *burden of proof* must be shifted. Factory owners should have to prove the safety of their waste products *before* they earn permits to dump. As it is now, the burden is on the public (whose interests are frequently not represented in the chambers of power) to prove that their safety is jeopardized. Foolishly transferring a value from our legal thinking to our chemical thinking, we have for too long assumed that pollutants are "innocent until proven guilty." Nuclear radiation, DDT, thalidomide and now mercury should teach us that our thinking has been dangerously mistaken.

Postscript

In the process of preparing this work, we have asked many questions and, in turn, have been asked quite a few ourselves. One of the most disturbing queries came to us from a young housewife in Albuquerque. "How can you be sure," she asked, "that another pollutant, just as insidious and just as dangerous as mercury, isn't right now spreading through our environment undetected?"

We had no easy answer for her. There isn't one. We could only reply that there is, of course, no absolute assurance another "mercury," if you will, isn't threatening the environment and the public's health right now. Not just one more insidious and undetected pollutant, but two or 10 or even 100. A recent search of the literature, in fact, reveals there are scores of potentially hazardous substances on the loose in the U.S. environment: feedstocks, dyes, organic and inorganic chemicals, medicinals, metals, fuels, pesticides, plastics.

There wasn't time, then, to read our questioner even a partial list. So we offer it now, knowing that each of the substances listed urgently deserves a closer scrutiny than mercury received, and that given America's technological tendencies, there will undoubtedly be many, many more to come:

acetylene
asphalt
benzene
coal tar pitch
ethylene
isobutylene
naphtha
naphthalene
petroleum distillate
toluene
xylene
aniline
cyclohexanone
cyclohexanol
dichlorophenol
dinitrophenol
ethyl benzene
hexachlorobenzene
isophorone
nitrobenzene
phthalic anhydride
phenol
p-nitrophenol
pyridine
styrene
amiline dyes

methol
ammonium chloride
ammonium nitrate
boranes (boron hydrides)
boric acid
boride dusts
bromine
calcium
carbides
carbon sulfide
chloride
chlorine
cyanide
fluoride
halogens
hydrogen fluoride
hydrogen peroxide
hydrogen sulfide
iodine
magnesium
nitrates
ozone
phosphoric acid
phosphorus
potassium arsenite
potassium cyanide
selenium
silicic acid
silicon tetrafluoride
siliceous carbon
sodium chloride
sodium cyanide

sulfates
sulfides
sulfuric acid
super phosphate
tellurium
tricalcium phosphate
ammoniated mercury ointment
amphetamine
1, 1, 1-trifluoroethyl vinyl ether
arsenitic acid
dihydrostreptomycin
griseofulvin
hormones (in cosmetics)
neomycin
penicillin
polymyxin
salicylate
streptomycin
aluminum
aluminum chloride
aluminum fluoride
aluminum phosphide
antimony
antimony oxide
arsenic
arsenicals
arsenic trioxide
barium
beryllium
cadmium
cadmium oxide
chromates

chromium
chromium boride
chromium carbide
chromium compounds
cobalt carbide
copper
copper sulfate
ferrous sulfate
germanium
indium
inorganic arsenicals
iron
iron dextran
iron silicate
lead
lead dioxide
manganese
manganese dioxide
mercuric cyanide
molybdenum
nickel
nickel carbonyl
rare earths
rare earth nitrates
rare earth oxides
silver
tantalum
thallium
tin
trace metals
trialkylgermanium compounds
tungsten carbide

vanadium
zinc
zinc beryllium silicate
zinc sulfate
aliphatic aldehydes
aromatic hydrocarbons
aromatics
artik tuf-lava
asbestos
cement
coal and coke
cryolite
fiber glass
fluorspar
glass
hematite
heterocyclic hydrocarbons
kaolin
kerosene
mineral oil
nitro-olefins
olefins
paraffins
polycyclic hydrocarbons
silica
solvents
talc
acetaldehyde
acetone
acrolein
aerosol propellant
aldehyde

arsine
benz [a] anthracene
benzo (k) fluoranthene
benzotrichloride
benzopyrene
benzpyrene
bithionol
bitumen
2-bromo-chloro-1, 1, 1, - trifluoroethane
carbazoles
carbon disulfide
carbon tetrachloride
chlorobenzol
chlorobromomethane
chloroform
chlorophose
chloroprene
delta amino-laevulinic acid
1, 1-dimethylhydrazine
dimethyldydrazine (UDMH)
dimethylsulfoxide
dinitroorthocresol
epoxide
ethyl mercaptan
ethylene glycol
ethylene glycol dinitrate
ethylene oxide
ethylenimine
fluorenthene
fluorocarbons
formaldehyde
freon

furfural
furfuramide
hairspray
hexamethylenediamino
lactone
mercaptans
methane diisocyanate
methane
menthanol
methyl nitrite
methylene-bis- (4 phenylisocyanate)
N, N'-di (acetoacetyl) -o-tolidine
neoprene
N-ethylethylenimine
nitroethylene
nitroglycerin
3-nitro-3-hexene
1-nitro-1-propene
pentachlorophenol
peroxyacetal nitrate (PAN)
peroxy compounds
phenylbutazone
phosgene
polytetrafluorethylene
polytrifluorochloroethylene
simazine
tetrachloroethylene
tetraethyl lead
tetramethyl lead
thorotrast
1, 1, 1-trichloroethane
trichloroethylene

tridymite
triethyleneglycol
triphenyltin acetate
toluene diisocyanate
agrosan GN
aldrin
bayluscide
bis-ethylmercury phosphate
chlordane
chlorophenothane DDT (DDE, TDE)
coumaphos (Co-Ral)
2-4-D
DDVP
dieldrin
dimethoate
endrin
guthion
heptachlor expoxide
heptachlor
ICI
lindane
malathion
mercury dicyandiamide
molluscicide
NaPCP
organic phosphate pesticides
organochlorine insecticides
parathion
pralidoximes
rogor
sudan
tetraethyl pyrophosphate (TEPP)

tetrachlorophenol
thiram
cellulose
styrene (vinyl benzene)
ABS
detergents
LAS
THE END?

Appendices

Table of Weights and Measures

Levels of mercury higher than natural background levels are assumed to be human contributions to the environment, or pollution. As we talk about background levels, against which we measure pollution, we need to arm ourselves with a few numerical ideas.

We are talking about *extremely small* amounts of mercury. For example, we speak of nanograms of mercury, which are billionths of a gram.

There are 454 grams to a pound, so a gram doesn't weigh much to begin with. A nanogram is 1/1,000,000,000 gram or 10^{-9} gram, or 0.035/1,000,000,000 of an ounce.

When we speak of mercury in the air we talk of nanograms of mercury per cubic meter of air, expressed ng/m^3. A cubic meter of air is about 1⅓ cubic yards.

When we speak of mercury in soil or water or in aquatic sediments we ordinarily speak of nanograms per gram or parts per billion (ng/g or ppb).

When we speak of mercury in fish or game birds we ordinarily talk in much larger quantities (though they're still microscopic). Because animals and fish concentrate mercury in their bodies, when describing wildlife pollution we usually speak of milligrams (thousandths of a gram) of mercury per kilogram (1,000 grams) of body weight or mg/kg. Mg/kg is the equivalent of parts per million, ppm.

Important Mercury Numbers
One pound equals 454 grams
1 kilogram (kg) equals 1,000 grams or 2.2 pounds
1 milligram (mg) equals 1/1,000 of a gram
1 microgram (μg) equals 1/1,000,000 of a gram
1 nanogram (ng) equals 1/1,000,000,000 of a gram

If you have	and you want your answer to be in	multiply by
μg/m³	ng/m³	1,000
μg/g	ng/g	1,000
mg/kg	ppm	1*
mg/kg	ng/g	1,000
mg/m³	ng/m³	1,000,000
ng/g	mg/kg	0.001
ng/g	ppb	1*
ppb	ppm	0.001
ppb	ng/g	1*
ppm	ppb	1,000
ppm	mg/kg	1*

* In other words, they're equal.

Two other measures of mercury may be encountered by citizens trying to find out about quicksilver pollution. For measuring mercury in water, the reader may occasionally see the term micrograms per liter (μg/l). Since a liter of water weighs approximately 1,000 gm., the unit of measure μg/l can be considered approximately equal to ppb.

Among air measurements the reader may encounter the unit μg/kg, or micrograms per kilogram. Since a cubic meter of air weighs roughly 1,000 grams, the unit μg/kg is roughly equal to ppb.

The Industrial Uses of Mercury

Here is a brief description of the important industrial uses of mercury. The industries are ranked here by size of 1969 consumption, the larger ones first:

- *Electrolytic preparation of chlorine and caustic soda (sodium hydroxide)* (increasing use)

  1959 consumption   *1969 consumption*

     442,928 pounds   1,574,720 pounds

  This is the largest and fastest-growing industrial use of mercury in the United States. Using mercury as the cathode in an electrolytic process, two basic chemicals can be formed: chlorine gas and caustic soda (sodium hydroxide).

  It was the rayon industry that first demanded mercury-grade caustic soda, which is of high purity. Rayon, or "artificial silk" as it was once known, came into use in the United States in 1911. The Viscose

Company that year produced 362,544 pounds of the synthetic yarn. By 1920, rayon production had sky-rocketed to 10,125,000 pounds. Between 1922 and 1940, production increased at an amazing 22 percent per year. Caustic soda production by the so-called mercury-cell method increased accordingly. Each ton of caustic soda "consumes" (and ultimately returns to the environment) between 0.5 and 1.0 pounds of mercury. Since the 1940s the biggest industrial user of mercury-grade caustic soda has been the aluminum industry, followed by the glass, paper, petroleum and detergent industries.

Chlorine gas produced by mercury cells in 1969 totaled about 8,000 tons per day from about 35 U.S. installations. Half of all chlorine gas goes into plastics manufacturing. For each ton of chlorine produced, the chlor-alkali industry in 1969 introduced 0.5 pounds of mercury to the environment.

- *Electrical apparatus* (increasing use)
  1959 consumption   *1969 consumption*
  676,780 pounds   1,417,400 pounds

The electrical apparatus industry finds mercury highly useful because of its physical characteristics. For example, "silent" light switches for home use are nothing but a small glass tube containing a little puddle of silver mercury. When you flip the switch "on," the bead of mercury scurries from one end of the glass tube to the other, where it now conducts electricity between two electrical contacts implanted through the wall of the glass tube. Moreover, mercury vapor finds use in neon tube lights, in arc rectifiers, in the bright, bluish highway lights found now in many municipalities, in transistor radio batteries and in fluorescent lights.

- *Paint* (increasing use)

1959 consumption	*1969 consumption*
Anti-fouling paint:	
75,468 pounds	18,544 pounds
Mildew-proofing paint:	
191,596 pounds	720,936 pounds

  Anti-fouling paints (which resist growth of seaweeds and barnacles) increasingly employ nonmercury compounds, but mildew-proofing paints (especially latex paints) increasingly employ mercury compounds. Mildew-proof paint finds use in almost any damp location—in ships, in shower rooms, in laundries, in swimming pool areas, in basements, in seashore homes. Latex paints find use everywhere.

- *Industrial controls* (increasing use)

1959 consumption	*1969 consumption*
468,464 pounds	530,556 pounds

  Because it conducts electricity so well, and because it is liquid, and because it is so heavy ($13\frac{1}{2}$ times the weight of water), mercury finds wide use in industrial control devices: thermometers, manometers, and many types of pressure gauges.

- *Dental preparations* (increasing use)

1959 consumption	*1969 consumption*
138,928 pounds	232,028 pounds

  Silver and gold fillings, mostly.

- *Catalysts* (increasing use)

1959 consumption
73,340 pounds

1969 consumption
224,808 pounds

Mercury serves in many chemical reactions as a catalyst, an agent that gets the reaction going. Mercury serves as catalyst in the production of several kinds of plastic, the most important being urethane and polyvinyl chloride (PVC).

PVC is the single most widely used plastic product in the world. PVC is used in phonograph records, printing plates, pencil barrels, toothbrush handles, bottles (especially cosmetics containers), ice-cube trays, pipe, pipe fittings, valve parts and siding for industrial buildings, to name only a few "unplasticized" PVC products.

Plasticized PVC—the same substance with an added agent to make it flexible—is found in rainwear, shower curtains, tablecloths, draperies, refrigerator bowl covers, baby pants, auto seat covers, belts, handbags, suspenders, wallets, upholstery for furniture, floor coverings (so-called vinyl tile, for example), tubing, hose, weather stripping, wire insulation, toys, buttons, grommets, gaskets and flashlight lenses.

Discovered in 1835, PVC was never manufactured commercially until 1927. Twenty years later, PVC production stood at 100 million pounds. Eight years later production hit 500 million pounds. And in 1969 production reached 2,978,503,000 pounds of PVC.

- *Agriculture* (decreasing use)

1959 consumption
243,352 pounds

1969 consumption
204,364 pounds

Since 1914, American and European farmers have dipped seed in mercury compounds to protect the seed against microorganisms for the first few days after planting. The practice became widespread throughout the world during the 1940s.

- *General laboratory use* (increasing use)

1959 consumption	*1969 consumption*
84,360 pounds	155,116 pounds

  Industrial, commercial and hospital laboratories use mercury in instruments and as a catalyst for chemical preparations. Technicians "fix" (preserve) biological samples using mercury. When finished, they incinerate the mercury or flush it.

- *Pharmaceutical*s (decreasing use)

1959 consumption	*1969 consumption*
130,492 pounds	55,024 pounds

  Mercury has been used for its germ-killing properties (to treat certain skin diseases, for example) since at least 400 B.C. When syphilis was finally recognized as a specific disease in 1495, mercury immediately came into widespread use against it.

  The biggest single pharmaceutical use of mercury today is as a diuretic, especially in treating patients suffering congestive heart failure. This use is decreasing. Other common pharmaceuticals containing mercury are contraceptives, vaginal douches and suppositories. Mercury added to many body and hand lotions prevents growth of bacteria inside the container. Remember mercurochrome? It was a mercury-based germ-killer.

- *Paper and pulp industry* (decreasing use)
  1959 consumption   *1969 consumption*
  331,360 pounds   42,408 pounds
  Mercury compounds prevent growth of green slime on paper-making equipment and prevent growth of mold and bacteria on pulp during months of damp storage. Heavy use of mercurials by the paper industry dropped off drastically in 1965 after a ruling by the Food and Drug Administration that no mercury residues could appear in paper food containers. But today, mercury dumped 10 to 30 years ago by paper mills is still polluting waterways and fish.

- *Amalgamation and purification of metals* (decreasing use)
  1959 consumption   *1969 consumption*
  20,140 pounds   14,820 pounds
  One of mercury's peculiar properties is its ability to bond itself to almost all the other common metals except iron and platinum. The resulting fusion creates an "amalgam" of mercury and the other metal. Zinc and aluminum, among others, can be purified to a very high degree by amalgamation and subsequent separation by electrolysis.

A State-by-state Pollution Survey

The following state-by-state survey is based on inter-
views with officials in all 50 states. From the information one strong conclusion can be drawn: State officials
need more data on the hazards of mercury pollution,
and on analytic techniques for sampling an environment. At present, ignorance prevails. (Only one state,
New York, has adequately surveyed its environment to
date, and there are specialists who question the adequa-
cy of sampling technique even in New York's case.)

In Swedish practice, the standard measure of mercury pollution in aquatic environments is a neutron activation analysis of the muscle tissue of the fresh-water
pike *(Esox lucius)*, particularly a pike weighing about
1 kilogram (2.2 pounds). Old, large fish generally contain disproportionately higher levels of mercury than
young, small fish; standardization of size of samples is
therefore important.

Standardization of species is also important because

differing species accumulate mercury in their bodies in differing amounts, even though they're exposed to the same aquatic environment. Generally speaking, the fish that are higher on the food chain contain more mercury than fish of equal age and weight lower on the food chain. Examples of fish high on the food chain are: walleye *(Stizostedion vitreum,* known informally as the walleyed pike or walleyed perch) ; pike *(Esox lucius,* also known as *Esox estor);* and yellow perch *(Perca flavescens).*

As Victor Lambou at the Environmental Protection Agency puts it, "The testing that has gone on so far has found the minimum amount of mercury we'll find if we look further. Especially in the first few months of testing, many analysts lost much of the mercury they were trying to test for, because they didn't know how volatile the stuff was. The mercury they've managed to find represents a minimum level; they'll find more as they look further."

The reader will note that, for some states in this survey, specific industries are listed by name. These companies were identified in government reports as known sources of mercury discharge as of September 1970. The waters receiving mercury discharge are also identified.

● *ALABAMA*

Mercury Source	*Receiving Waters*
Diamond Shamrock, Muscle Shoals, Ala.	Pond Creek to Tennessee River
Olin Mathieson Chem., McIntosh, Ala.	Tombigbee River
Stauffer Chem. Co., Axis, Ala.	Mobile River

Some 51,000 acres of prime water closed to commercial fishing at estimated loss of $1 million in 1970. Additional losses, because of warnings to sport fishermen and subsequent drop in tourism and recreational spending, perhaps as high as $5 million.

Commercial fishing closed in the Tombigbee, Mobile, and Tennessee rivers. Sport fishermen warned to release their catch from the Tombigbee River up to Jackson Dam, and throughout the Mobile, Tensaw, and Tennessee rivers.

● *ALASKA*

Seals, which pick up mercury from the fish they eat and concentrate it in their livers, exhibited levels as high as an amazing 172 ppm in samples (of 50 seals) from the Pribilof Islands.

Alaska has not tested its fresh-water fish. The Bureau of Commercial Fisheries is surveying hair seals along the Alaska coast to determine extent of pollution, which is feared to be considerable.

Cinnabar mines up the Yukon River may be polluting the Yukon delta, game officials report.

● *ARIZONA*

Mercury Source	*Receiving Waters*
General Mercury Corp., Tempe, Arizona	Ground water (via leach field)
Pioneer Paint & Varnish Co., Tucson, Arizona	Santa Cruz River

The livers of 38 percent of 64 quail tested showed levels above 0.5 ppm, but breast tissue revealed none above 0.2 ppm.

Results on fish not yet available.

- *ARKANSAS*

Abandoned cinnabar mines have been flooded with water by Army Corps of Engineers dams, and may be contaminating fish on the western side of the state. Further checking is underway.

Arkansas monitors all waters entering or leaving its state borders and hasn't yet found mercury pollution above background levels.

- *CALIFORNIA*

Mercury Source	*Receiving Waters*
Garrett-Callahan Co., Millbrae, Calif.	Millbrae sewage treatment plant to San Francisco Bay
Quicksilver Prod., San Francisco, Calif.	City of San Francisco sewage treatment plant to San Francisco Bay

Flesh of pheasant has been tested, revealing levels as high as 4.7 ppm. Flesh of fish found to contain up to 1.29 ppm.

A federal-state mercury task force in California has warned pregnant women not to eat fish from San Francisco Bay and certain lakes.

Striped bass seem particularly contaminated, especially specimens larger than four pounds. Affected areas include San Francisco Bay, the Merced River, the Sacramento River, the Feather River, Carquinez Straits, and the San Joaquin River. Clear Lake and Lake Berryessa contain fish contaminated up to 1.25 ppm.

- *COLORADO*

State game and fish authorities report mercury levels of 0.04 to 0.6 ppm in pheasant, and up to 2.0 ppm in pheasant eggs. Mercury levels in sage grouse range from 0.04 up to an alarming 16.0 ppm.

Inexplicably, one chub low on the food chain in Colorado's part of Navajo Lake Reservoir contained 8.9 ppm. Colorado officials are "stunned" by this news because there is no known source of mercury in Colorado.

Brown trout in Navajo Lake average 0.9 ppm mercury in their edible flesh.

● *CONNECTICUT*

Bass in the Housatonic River and yellow perch in the Connecticut River occasionally show levels as high as 0.69 ppm and 0.78 ppm respectively, but state health officials minimize any talk of hazard.

Sea fish, such as striped bass along the edge of Long Island Sound, haven't been tested, though health authorities say they would expect to find more mercury there than elsewhere in Connecticut.

● *DELAWARE*

Mercury Source	*Receiving Waters*
Diamond Shamrock,	Delaware River
Delaware City, Dela.	

Samples of fish and water in the Delaware River reported below the "FDA limit of 0.5 ppm"—according to a report to federal authorities which apparently fails to take account of the significant difference between the FDA's standard for fish (0.5 ppm, or 500 ppb) and the Bureau of Water Hygiene's drinking water standard (0.005 ppm, or 5 ppb). While Delaware authorities were filing their report, FWQA investigators and the Justice Department were accusing Diamond Shamrock of polluting the Delaware River with mercury.

- *FLORIDA*

Florida officials say their state is not polluted by mercury. They are planning to test blue crabs soon. They have completed tests of water and riverbed sediments without finding anything. They are not anticipating finding polluted fish or shellfish.

- *GEORGIA*

Mercury Source	*Receiving Waters*
Olin Mathieson Chem. Corp. Augusta, Ga.	Savannah River

Savannah River, from New Savannah Dam to Highway 12, closed; New Brunswick estuary also closed to sport and commercial fishermen.

- *HAWAII*

Game and fish authorities report they have no laboratory facilities. They don't expect to find any mercury anyway, so they are not looking for it.

- *IDAHO*

After Alberta, Canada, alerted Idaho authorities to danger, subsequent investigation revealed mercury in the breast muscle of pheasant, ranging in concentrations from zero up to 7 ppm, with one sample as high as 15 ppm. Idaho authorities thereupon issued a poster, to be displayed wherever guns or ammunition are sold, warning hunters not to eat the pheasant they bag.

Idaho fishing waters seem to be polluted despite the absence of industrial users of mercury. Analysis of 160 fish of 19 species reveals 19.3 percent with levels above the FDA guideline of 0.5 ppm. Highest contamination found to date is 1.7 ppm in one squawfish in Hells Canyon on the Snake River. What's more, 45 percent of channel catfish and 39 percent of yellow perch seem to be contaminated well above the FDA guideline.

- *ILLINOIS*

Catfish containing up to 0.44 ppm has been sampled in state waters; white bass at 0.2 ppm; carp at 0.2 ppm. Sampling, however, has only just begun.

- *INDIANA*

No stream closures due to mercury contamination, but fish and game officials note that fewer fishermen participated in the 1970 fishing season than in the previous year—despite increased fishing opportunities within the state.

Indiana has only recently established a sampling schedule. Twenty-five samples from Lake Michigan so far show no levels above 0.5 ppm; 10 tested pheasant contained up to 0.46 ppm in their feathers (through which birds excrete mercury), but in their edible flesh none tested higher than 0.058.

- *IOWA*

No mercury found so far in Iowa waters.

- *KANSAS*

  Federal tests for pesticides this past fall included mercury analysis for the first time. No results available yet.

- *KENTUCKY*

Mercury Source	*Receiving Waters*
Goodrich Chem. Co., Calvert City, Ky.	Tennessee River
Pennwalt Chem. Co., Calvert City, Ky.	Tennessee River

  Despite refusal of state officials to close certain streams to commercial fishing, the FDA announced that commercial fishing in Kentucky is as good as finished, that the interstate shipment of Kentucky fish is virtually banned. Tennessee River is contaminated below Kentucky Dam. A loss of at least $250,000 a year for commercial fishing in Kentucky Lake-Tennessee River area.

- *LOUISIANA*

Mercury Sources	*Receiving Waters*
Dow Chem. Co., Plaquemine, La.	Mississippi River
Monochem. Inc., Geismar, La.	Mississippi River
PPG Industries Lake Charles, La.	Bayou d'Inde
Wyandotte Chem., Geismar, La.	Mississippi River

  Calcasieu Lake closed to commercial fishing; sport fishermen warned there and on the Calcasieu River against eating their catch.

- *MAINE*

Mercury Source	*Receiving Waters*
International Mining & Chem. Co., Orrington, Maine	Penobscot River
Oxford Paper Co., Rumford, Maine	Androscoggin River

State fish and game officials "think" FDA officials tested Maine waters in one or two locations last year but they say they've seen no results.

Because Maine has so many paper mills, that state *especially* should be watching for fish contamination.

Despite assurances from paper mill owners that they now use no mercury, they most likely used tons of mercury up until the mid-1960s when many paper mills changed chemicals. Mercury pollution from the mid-1960s and earlier *still* contaminates our waters today because mercury sinks to the bottom, then starts moving slowly out through food chains.

- *MARYLAND*

Maryland fish and game officials appear reticent to discuss mercury pollution. Yet as early as 1960, public health officials reported shellfish in Chesapeake Bay contained mercury up to 2,000 ppb (2 ppm).

- *MASSACHUSETTS*

Fish in the Merrimack and Taunton rivers contain concentrations ranging from 0.17 to 1.21 ppm. In shellfish, mussels and clams in Taunton estuary, levels range from 0.3 to 0.47 ppm.

Massachusetts authorities checked fish at 10 sites

throughout the state and found fish contaminated by more than 0.5 ppm in 43 percent of the fish sampled.

- *MICHIGAN*

Mercury Source	*Receiving Waters*
General Electric Co., Edmore, Mich.	Cedar Lake to Pine River
Wyandotte Chem., Wyandotte, Mich.	Detroit River

Michigan has closed Lake St. Clair to commercial fishing. Fish from the lake contain up to 7.09 ppm in their flesh. Subsequent U.S. Department of Interior tests reveal levels from 0.01 to 1.76 ppm in waterfowl collected from Lake St. Clair.

Ducks from the Detroit River area contain up to 7.5 ppm in their livers, and up to 2.26 ppm in breast muscle. The Detroit River is said to be the most mercury-polluted body of water in America.

- *MINNESOTA*

Fish in 27 locations were tested. Excessive mercury was found in Lake Minewaska, Lake Mille Lacs, Otter Tail Lake, as well as in the Red River at Oslo, the Mississippi at Grand Rapids, the St. Louis estuary at Duluth, the Mississippi at Brainard and at Monticello, the Minnesota River at St. Peter, the Mississippi River between Springer Lake and Hastings, the St. Croix River at Taylor Falls.

- *MISSISSIPPI*

Pickwick Reservoir closed to commercial fishing. Levels in fish range from 0.05 to 1.14 ppm.

- *MISSOURI*
  No reports of mercury pollution.

- *MONTANA*
  Preliminary testing reveals excessive levels of mercury in suckers and trout from the Beaverhead River and drainage and at Grasshopper Creek, especially near the town of Dillon. Trout at the Dillon sewage outfall show levels up to 1.32 ppm.

  Some 67 percent of partridge in south central Montana contain mercury above the 0.5 ppm guideline. Partridge from other areas contain less, though still measurable, levels of mercury.

- *NEBRASKA*
  No results yet from a recent testing program.

- *NEVADA*
  Initial results of tests in the Truckee and Carson rivers promise discovery of contamination. Fish in both rivers are believed contaminated up to 1.1 ppm.

  Nevada has many natural deposits of mercury.

- *NEW HAMPSHIRE*
  Danger warnings were issued to fishermen on the Connecticut and Merrimack rivers because pickerel, yellow perch, smallmouth and largemouth bass were found to contain mercury above 0.5 ppm. Highest concentration recorded: 1.3 ppm.

  About 1,000 samples have been taken. Of these samples, 15 percent run above 0.5 ppm. In 25 of the state's ponds, 25 percent of the fish exceed 0.5 ppm.

- *NEW JERSEY*

Mercury Source	*Receiving Waters*
General Aniline & Film Corp., Linden, N.J.	Arthur Kill
Woodbridge Chem., Woodbridge, N.J.	Berrys Creek to Hackensack River

  Raritan Bay is closed to shellfishing because of mercury and a dozen other contaminants. Beyond this, New Jersey knows almost nothing about the parameters of its mercury problem. It was to begin testing in 1971.

- *NEW MEXICO*

  On October 15, 1970, fish and game authorities declared their state's biggest recreation lake, Elephant Butte Reservoir, on the Rio Grande River, contaminated. FDA analysis revealed mercury at the following levels: walleyed pike, 1.29 ppm; white bass, 0.91 ppm; channel catfish, 0.68 ppm; flathead catfish, 0.63 ppm.

  The state has now appropriated $80,000 emergency funds to discover the source of mercury and set up its own testing laboratory.

  The other major state water known to contain fish contaminated above the 0.5 ppm level is Navajo Lake on the Colorado-New Mexico border.

- *NEW YORK*

Mercury Sources	*Receiving Waters*
Allied Chemical Co., Buffalo, N.Y.	Buffalo River to Lake Erie

Allied Chemical Co., Solvay, N.Y.	Onondaga Lake
Chesebrough-Ponds, Inc., Faichney Inst., Watertown, N.Y.	Black River to Lake Ontario
Hooker Electrochem., Niagara Falls, N.Y.	Niagara Falls sewer system and Niagara River
Olin Mathieson Chem., Niagara Falls, N.Y.	Niagara River
Williams Gold Refining Co., Buffalo, N.Y.	City of Buffalo sewage treatment plant to Niagara River

Nearly 7,000 samples of fish flesh taken from New York waters resulted in the closure of sport-fishing on Onondaga Lake, a warning to fishermen not to eat their catch from Lake Champlain, Lake Erie, Lake Ontario, the Oswego River, the Niagara River and the St. Lawrence River. Saratoga Lake and Lake George are now believed to be contaminated as well.

The range of mercury levels found in fish by this, the single most extensive mercury search by any state, was 0.01 to 8.2 ppm, (10 ppb to 8,200 ppb). Range of mercury found in (treated) municipal drinking water: .0004 to .0040 ppm, (.4 ppb to 4 ppb).

● *NORTH CAROLINA*

Mercury Source	*Receiving Water*
Riegel Paper Co. Riegelwood, N.C.	Cape Fear River

Fairly extensive testing seems to reveal no measurable pollution in North Carolina's waters. Even the lower Cape Fear River seems free of mercury pollution, according to state game officials. Maybe.

● *NORTH DAKOTA*
Tests in Froelich Reservoir, Lake Ashtabula, Jamestown Reservoir, Spirit Wood Lake, Red River, Lake Sakakawea and Lake Oahe reveal contamination as high as 1 ppm in several species. No known source; airborne mercury suspected.

● *OHIO*

Mercury Sources	Receiving waters
Detrex Chem. Ind., Ashtabula, Ohio	Ditch to Lake Erie
General Electric Chem. Prod. Plant, Cleveland, Ohio	Lake Erie
NASA, Lewis Research Center Cleveland, Ohio	Rocky River
Reactive Metals, Inc., Ashtabula, Ohio	West Branch, Fields Brook to Fields Brook to Ashtabula River

The state of Ohio has sued Dow Chemical's Sarnia, Canada, plant for polluting Lake Erie, causing international complications which must be sorted out by the Supreme Court of the United States.

● *OKLAHOMA*
Preliminary tests reveal no pollution above background levels in either water or fish.

- *OREGON*

  Only about one of 10 pheasants sampled shows a level of mercury in breast muscle exceeding 0.5 ppm.

  On the Columbia, significant pollution has been discovered from the mouth of the Willamette River to St. Helena or below. In crayfish in the Columbia, mercury reaches 3.02 ppm, and in sturgeon it is up to 0.779 ppm.

  Bass in the Willamette, as well as trout, carp and bullheads, exceed the FDA guideline.

- *PENNSYLVANIA*

Mercury Source	*Receiving Waters*
Mallinckrodt Chem., Erie, Pa.	City of Erie sewage treatment plant to Lake Erie
NOSCO Plastics, Erie, Pa.	City of Erie sewage treatment plant to Lake Erie

  Lake Erie waters are clearly contaminated. Sport fishermen have been warned to release rainbow trout, coho salmon, walleye, drum, smallmouth bass and white bass. A few of each species show levels reaching a frightening 3.0 ppm.

- *RHODE ISLAND*

  Fresh-water fish haven't yet been tested. Of 38 lobsters tested from four areas, none exceeded the FDA guideline but lobsters from one area—Vetch Canyon, out near the edge of the continental shelf—came close.

- *SOUTH CAROLINA*
  Savannah River from Augusta to the coast is closed to commercial and sportfishing.

- *SOUTH DAKOTA*
  Angostura Reservoir and the Cheyenne River arm of Oahe Reservoir (40,000 acres, approximately) are suspected of being contaminated.

- *TENNESSEE*

Mercury Sources	*Receiving Waters*
Buckeye Cellulose, Memphis, Tenn.	Wolf River to Mississippi River
Buckman Labs., Memphis, Tenn.	Lateral sewer to Wold River interceptor to Mississippi River
Chapman Chem. Co., Memphis, Tenn.	Hon Connah Creek to Mississippi River
Olin Mathieson Chem., Charleston, Tenn.	Hiwassee River

  Pickwick Lake and the Tennessee River are closed to commercial fishing, and sport fishermen have been warned to throw back fish taken from those waters.

- *TEXAS*

Mercury Sources	*Receiving Waters*
Aluminum Co. of America, Point Comfort, Texas	Lavaca Bay
Diamond Shamrock Chem. Co., Deer Park, Texas	Houston Ship Channel

Monsanto Chem. Co.,	Galveston Bay
Texas City, Texas	
Tenneco Chem. Co.,	Houston Ship Channel
Pasadena, Texas	

Some 19,900 acres of Lavaca Bay are closed to commercial oyster fishing because of mercury. Fulvis tree ducks were found containing mercury above 0.5 ppm in two out of three samples.

● *UTAH*

Mercury Source	*Receiving Waters*
Hill Air Force Base,	North Davis County sewage
Ogden, Utah	treatment plant

Preliminary surveys of pheasant and fish show some contamination. Of 25 pheasant sampled, one contained mercury in breast tissue above 0.5 ppm.

Fish in Willard Bay Reservoir (Box Elder County) reveal walleyed pike contaminated up to an alarming 3.29 ppm. Of six walleyed pike sampled, none contained less than 0.91 ppm. Bass range from 0.35 ppm up to 1.0 ppm. Carp range from 0.59 ppm up to 1.21 ppm.

More tests are underway.

● *VERMONT*

Commercial fishing has been banned on Lake Champlain and Lake Memphremagog, and sport fishermen have been warned against eating their catch from those lakes. A total of 873 fish samples from 27 locations revealed levels of mercury ranging from 0.1 to 2.00 ppm.

Fish in Silver Lake, on a mountaintop accessible only by four-wheel-drive vehicle, contain levels above 0.5 ppm. Investigators are now looking for airborne mercury sources.

The ban on commercial fishing hurts no major businesses, but has severely restricted ice-fishing for hundreds, perhaps thousands, of Vermonters who pick up a few extra dollars that way to get through the winter. As usual, the poor suffer most from pollution.

● *VIRGINIA*

Mercury Source	*Receiving Waters*
Olin Mathieson Chem., Saltsville, Va.	North Fork, Holston River

The North fork of the Holston River, below Saltsville, is contaminated. Fishermen have been warned their catch may be dangerous.

● *WASHINGTON*

Mercury Sources	*Receiving Waters*
Georgia-Pacific, Bellingham, Wash.	Puget Sound
Weyerhaeuser Co., Longview, Wash.	Columbia River

Livers of fur seals are contaminated at very high levels: 60.7 to 72.6 ppm.

Fresh-water fish appear uncontaminated. Columbia River raw water averages 1 ppb.

Washington has many abandoned cinnabar mines that produced mercury for the manufacture of explosives (mercury fulminate) during World War II and the war in Korea.

- *WEST VIRGINIA*

Mercury Source	Receiving Waters
Allied Chemical Co., Moundsville, W. Va	Ohio River
PPG Industries, Natrium, W. Va.	Ohio River
Westinghouse, Fairmont, W. Va.	Monongahela River

The Monongahela and Ohio rivers are severely polluted. Commercial fishermen have been "advised" by governor to cease operations. Sport fishermen "advised" not to eat their catch from these two rivers.

- *WISCONSIN*

Mercury Source	Receiving Waters
Wyandotte Chem., Port Edwards, Wisc.	Wisconsin River

Citizens are advised not to eat fish more than once a week from 430-mile stretch of the Wisconsin River where mercury levels are as high as 4.62 ppm in fish flesh.

- *WYOMING*

Pheasant in Wyoming average 0.2 to 0.25 ppm; one out of 30 birds tested contained up to 0.6 ppm. Results on fish are not yet available.

Workplace Standards

The U.S. government has set no TLV (threshold limit value) for mercury. A private organization, the American Conference of Governmental and Industrial Hygienists (ACGIH) sets such standards in the United States.

Prior to 1968 the internationally recognized MAC value (maximum allowable concentration, the international equivalent of the value expressed in America as a threshold limit value) for mercury was the same as the ACGIH value.

However, in 1968 a group of 16 international specialists in industrial hygiene and mercury met at the Karolinska Institute, Stockholm, to set a new international MAC value.

The new international recommendation emerging from the 1968 Karolinska meeting asks that mercury be divided into three categories, according to its toxicity. The most toxic compounds, primarily methyl mercury, are so dangerous that the Karolinska group refused to set an unequivocal numerical level of concentration for methyl mercury in workplace air. The group recommended instead that workers exposed to methyl mercury have their blood periodically analyzed for mercury content, and they recommended that the concentration of mercury in workers' blood *never* be allowed to exceed 10 micrograms mercury per 100 milliliters blood. "This blood level is not likely to be reached with daily intake of 100 micrograms mercury in the form of methyl mercury . . . this intake corresponds to an average air concentration of 0.01 mg/m³ [10,000 ng/m³]," concluded the Karolinska group.

For elemental mercury vapor the Karolinska group recommended 50,000 ng/m³ maximum allowable concentration for workplace air breathed during an eighthour shift.

For inorganic mercury salts, and phenyl mercury and methoxyethyl mercury salts (the latter two being organic compounds) , the Karolinska group recommended ambient air concentrations not exceeding 100,000 ng/m³. The Karolinska group noted that the organic mercury salts seem to be just as toxic as elemental mercury vapor but the salts are usually encountered in the work environment as aerosols, which are not absorbed by the lungs as efficiently as elemental mercury vapor. Therefore the group set a higher allowable concentration for the inorganic salts and the two organics.

Three American scientists sat on the international panel at Karolinska Institute in 1968: Dr. Leonard J. Goldwater, Dr. Thomas W. Clarkson, and Dr. Ralph G. Smith.

The ACGIH has recently announced that it intends to tighten its mercury standards. The new ACGIH standard is going to recognize two mercury groups, the alkyl mercury compounds, and all other mercury compounds. For the alkyl mercury compounds the new ACGIH standard is going to be the same as its present one: 10,000 ng/m³.

For all other mercury compounds besides the alkyl mercurials, the new ACGIH recommendation will be 50,000 ng/m³, just half the present ACGIH standard.

According to information available from the federal government (specifically a literature review on airborne mercury carried out by Litton Industries, Inc., for the National Air Pollution Control Administration and published by HEW in October, 1969), the proposed international mercury standards are not tight.

In the Litton study we read of Russian lab experiments in which white rats inhaled air artificially polluted with elemental mercury vapor at levels as low as 2,000 to 5,000 ng/m^3. These rats accumulated mercury in their kidneys, liver, heart and brain, and they "exhibited pathomorphological changes and *disturbances of the functional activity of the higher nerve centers.*" (Emphasis added.)

Thus, rats suffer nervous system damage at air concentrations 10 to 20 times lower than the numbers recommended by the Karolinska group. Workmen on the job can hardly feel protected by the Karolinska recommendations.

The matter of worker safety around mercury demands careful, prompt attention by scientists (and lawmakers and union officials) operating completely independently of industry. Mercury is too serious a business for American workers to settle for less. Only the tightest standards vigorously and strictly enforced can protect the nation's work force. Appropriate penalties and sanctions need to be applied.

The Karolinska group made one final observation worth stressing here: "The group finds it advisable," said their report, "that women of child-bearing age should not have exposure to any alkyl mercury compounds occupationally."

ment of Health, Education and Welfare, Office of Technical Information and Publications, National Air Pollution Control Administration, 1033 Wade Ave., Raleigh, N.C. 27605. Price not available. Another source for this publication is: National Technical Information Service, Springfield, Virginia 22151. $ 3.00.

   Literature on air-borne mercury reviewed.

Swedish Royal Commission on Natural Resources (ed.). *Oikos* [Acta Oecologica Scandinavica] Supplementum 9 (1967) / The Mercury Problem/ Symposium concerning mercury in the environment held at Wenner-Gren Center, Stockholm, January 24–26, 1966. Published by: Munsksgaard International Booksellers and Publishers, Prags Boulevard 47, Copenhagen S, Denmark. $12.75 U.S.

   A goldmine of early information.

United States Geological Survey. *Mercury in the Environment/ Geological Survey Professional Paper 713* (Washington, D.C., 1970). Available from Superintendent of Documents, U.S. Government Printing Office, Washington, D.C. 20402. $ .70.

   An anthology of 11 essays, all by government scientists. Very useful. Bibliographies. Tables. Charts.

U.S. Tariff Commission. Mercury (Quicksilver), Report on Investigation No. 32, Under Section 332 of the Tariff Act of 1930 (Nov., 1958). Available from: U.S. Tariff Commission, Washington, D.C., 20436. No charge.

U.S. Tariff Commission. Mercury (Quicksilver), Report to the Congress on Investigation No. 332-32 (Supplemental), Under Section 332 of the Tariff Act of 1930 (May, 1962). Available from: U.S. Tariff Commission, Washington, D.C. 20436.

   Heavy going, but both are worthy catalogs on the mercury industry.

Wallace, Robin A., William Fulkerson, Wilbur D. Shults, and William S. Lyon. *Mercury in the Environment/*

The Human Element (Oak Ridge, Tenn., Jan., 1971).
Available as Publication No. ORNL NSF-EP-1 from
Oak Ridge National Laboratory, Oak Ridge, Tenn.
37830.

   The best short summary available to date; bibli-
ography.

Wood, J. M. "Environmental Pollution by Mercury," to
   appear later in 1971 in Robert C. Badger (ed.), *Ad-
   vances in Environmental Science,* Vol. II, by John
   Wiley & Sons, Inc., 605 Third Ave., New York, N.Y.
   10016.

About the Sierra Club

The Sierra Club, founded in 1892 by John Muir, has consistently devoted itself to the study and protection of America's scenic resources and wild places. Sierra Club publications are part of the nonprofit effort the club carries on as a public trust. There are chapters in all parts of the United States. Participation is invited in the club's program to enjoy and preserve wilderness, wildlife, and a quality environment for all men, for all time.

The Sierra Club
Mills Tower
San Francisco, California 94104
Please enroll me as a member of the Sierra Club.

Name_____

Address_____

City, state, zip _____

   Dues: $5 admission, plus $12 (regular membership), $6 (spouse), or $5 (junior member under 21).

I enclose _____.

Another Sierra Club Battlebook:

Oil on Ice
Alaskan Wilderness at the Crossroads

The issue in Alaska centers on an estimated 100 billion barrels of oil buried beneath the frigid landscape of America's last great wilderness. But the issue raises a question: What effect will the extraction of that treasure have on Alaska's fragile environment, particularly if the oil is transported to market through an equally fragile trans-Alaska pipeline? *Oil on Ice* seeks to answer that question, and many others. Before the questions become academic.

The author of *Oil on Ice* is Tom Brown, crack legislative correspondent and environmental writer for the *Anchorage Daily News*. The editor is Richard Pollak, a former *Newsweek* writer and frequent contributor to national magazines. Two weeks after publication, readers had snapped up the entire first printing. Anyone who is concerned about what happens to Alaska should read *Oil on Ice*. Before Alaska becomes academic, too.

160 pages, with map.
At your bookstore, $1.95.